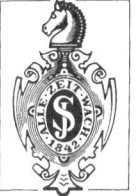

Judit Daróczy

The Dermal Lymphatic Capillaries

With 174 Figures

Springer-Verlag
Berlin Heidelberg New York London Paris Tokyo

Dr. Judit Daróczy
Kàllai Èva Hospital
of State's Hospital Stephan
Kun n. 4
1081 Budapest, Hungary

Library of Congress Cataloging-in-Publication Data
Daróczy, Judit. *The dermal lymphatic capillaries.* Bibliography: p. Includes index. 1. Skin – Lymphatics –
Ultrastructure. I. Title. [DNLM: 1. Lymphatic System. WH 700 D224d]   QM197.D37   1988   611'.42 88-22421
ISBN-13: 978-3-642-73482-3   e-ISBN-13: 978-3-642-73480-9
DOI: 10.1007/ 978-3-642-73480-9

© Springer-Verlag Berlin Heidelberg 1988
Softcover reprint of the hardcover 1st edition 1988

Typesetting: Appl, Wemding
2127/3145–543210 Printed on acid-free paper

Preface

The importance of the lymphatic system has been known for a long time. It was therefore surprising to learn that the status of dermal lymphatics, under both normal and pathological conditions of man, had been largely neglected to date, particularly with respect to their ultrastructure. Moreover, the existing information is incomplete, relating only to narrow segments of the skin, and it is controversial.

This monograph represents an effort to overcome some of the existing deficiencies in the area of the structure (with emphasis on ultrastructure) of lymphatic capillaries. It is an account of our experience in the evaluation of dermal lymphatics in normal, edematous, and some other pathological conditions in man and in experimental animals.

It is hoped that this information will prove useful for other investigators as a basis for evaluation of the structural and functional status of dermal lymphatics under a wide variety of pathological conditions. To the best of my knowledge, much of the information on the ultrastructure of the dermal lymphatics presented herein is new.

This work would not have been possible without the inspiration of Prof. Dr. I. ANTON-LAMPRECHT, Head of the Institute for Ultrastructure Research of the Skin, Department of Dermatology of the University of Heidelberg, Federal Republic of Germany.

I gratefully acknowledge the generous support of the Alexander von Humboldt Foundation of Germany, which enabled me to carry out a major portion of the work upon which the monograph was based, in Heidelberg.

Budapest, August 1988   Dr. JUDIT DARÓCZY

Table of Contents

Materials and Methods

Human Material. Normal and pathological skin of the forearm, lower leg, and back were studied. The biopsies were taken from the following disorders (under local anaesthesia): lymphedema, hyperkeratosis, atrophic skin lesions, ichthyosis vulgaris, pityriasis rubra pilaris, toxicoderma, lymphangioma circumscriptum, pseudo-Kaposi's sarcoma, Kaposi's sarcoma, porphyria cutanea tarda, hyalinosis cutis et mucosae, lichen amyloidosus, lymphangitis carcinomatosa.

Experimental Material. Canine: Male and female canines weighing 15–25 kg were used for this study. Lymphedema was produced by the ligation of the lymphatic trunk in the femoral region (SOLTI 1986). Skin biopsies were taken from the normal hind limbs and from the operated extremities of the animals after 10–14 days they were operated. *Rat:* Wistar rats weighing 150–200 g were injected i.v. with 50 g/100 g body weight of native ferritin (dialysed, Nutritional Biochemicals Corporation,

Cleveland, Ohio) 20 min before being killed. Tissue samples from the upper and lower paws were taken from the animals under ether anesthesia. Blocks of skin from the upper and lower paws were fixed in KARNOVSKY's fixative (KARNOVSKY 1965) and postfixed in OsO_4 with lanthanum according to SHEA (1971). The paraffin embedded materials were stained with hematoxylin and eosin, orcein, GÖMÖRI's silver impregnation, and WEIGERT's resorcin-fuchsin staining. The samples for electron microscopic studies were fixed by immersion using KARNOVSKY's fixative and postfixed with OsO_4 (DARÓCZY and HÜTTNER 1978). The tissues were treated for 2 h with uranyl acetate en bloc and embedded in Epon. The semithin, toluidine-blue stained sections were reviewed by light microscopy. The thin sections were cut with Reichert UmO_2 ultrotome and examined either unstained or following uranyl acetate and lead citrate staining with JEM 7A and Philips EM-600 microscopes.

1 The Lymphatic Tree

The phylogenesis and comparative anatomy are described for the large lymphatic vessels and trunks (TÖNDURY and KUBIK 1972). The lymphatic tree (human) can be grouped into three categories.

1.1 Lymphatic Trunk

The lymphatic trunk represents the thoracic duct and empties into the great veins of the neck. The vessel contains valves and the wall consists of three distinct tunics: (a) the tunica intima, comprising endothelial layer surrounded by basal lamina, (b) the tunica media, consisting of alternating layers of smooth muscle cells and collagen and elastic fibers, and (c) the tunica adventitia, composed of collagen and elastic fibers intermingled with fibroblasts, in addition to nerve bundles and small blood vessels.

1.2 Lymphatic Collecting Vessels

The lymphatic capillaries empty into the lymphatic collecting vessels. The collecting vessels are punctured with lymph nodes. They lie in the mid and deep dermis, especially at the junction of the dermis with the subcutaneous tissue and in the septa of fat lobules. The form of their luminal cross sections depends on the phase of their activity. The vessels can be oval, round, cruciform, or star-shaped.

The collecting vessels have three wall layers: beneath the endothelial tunica intima the smooth muscle cells create the tunica media. The muscle cells are intermingled with collagen and elastic fibers. At the basis region of the valves the smooth muscle layer is lacking, but it

is prominent along the wall segments between the valves. The elastic fibers do not form an elastic membrane, but rather a loose network accompanied by fibroblasts in the tunica adventitia (OEHMKE 1968; LEAK 1972a). Unmyelinated nerve bundles can be present. The collecting lymphatic vessels contain valves and they have a well-developed basal lamina. The endothelial junctions are tightly closed; thus, large molecules and cells can not escape from the vessels but water and small molecules may migrate outward.

1.3 Lymphatic Capillaries

The smallest lymphatic vessels have been termed "terminal lymphatics", "small lymphatics", or "initial lymphatics". The different terminologies are misleading; like the small blood vessels they are classified as capillaries. They contain valves, and the permeable wall consists of endothelial cells. The presence of endothelial gaps is common, and a continuous basal lamina is lacking. In the perivascular interstitium the elastic fibers are intermingled with collagen fibers and with the microfilaments running directly to the abluminal membrane of the capillary endothelial cells.

The lymphatic plexus begins in the dermis as blind tubes in the dermal papillae; these join with neighboring capillaries to form the superficial lymphatic plexus. The deep lymphatic plexus is composed of lymphatics of varying caliber, which are situated in the deeper layers of the dermis (ZSDANOV 1952).

PFLEGER (1964a) described postcapillary lymphatics which were situated at the cutis-subcutis boundary. In their wall, smooth muscle cells could be demonstrated.

The term "dermal lymphatic capillary" represents a lymph vessel lacking continuous basal lamina and smooth muscle cells in its wall.

The term "prelymphatics" represents the path of least resistance through the connective tissue directed toward the lymphatics. They are preformed paths in the vicinity of lymphatics (CASLEY-SMITH and SIMS 1976). The lymphatic lumen contains flocculent material which appears medium dense under the electron microscope and it is interpreted as being protein-rich lymph. This flocculent material is observed in the adjacent perilymphatic areas as well.

2 How to Demonstrate Lymphatic Capillaries

The demonstration of the lymphatic drainage system and the lymphatic capillaries represents a problem because of the vulnerability of the walls of lymph vessels.

Various techniques have been used to visualize the lymphatic vessels:

1. The blocking of the lymph flow leads to lymphostasis, with dilatation of the vascular lumina up to the capillary endings, which are viewed microscopically.
2. Injection of a lymph-specific dye, such as patent blue, that appears electively in the lymph vessels demonstrates branches of the skin lymphatics.
3. Radiological lymphangiography using contrast medium makes the lymphatic vessels visible (KINMONTH 1952).
4. Subepidermal injection of a non-ionic water-soluble contrast medium is used in indirect lymphangiography to produce opacity of lymphatic capillaries and collecting vessels in the skin (PARTSCH 1983).
5. Fluorescence lymphography requires special equipment (BOLLINGER 1981).
6. Isotopic lymphangiography (LINDEMAYR et al. 1984) involves injection of isotope-labeled protein subepidermally, after which the clearance of the protein from the interstitium is monitored (ELLIS et al. 1970).

Injection techniques carry the risk of rupturing the walls of the lymphatic capillaries. In this way the interstitial spaces or the prelymphatics may be filled, and these could suggest the presence of lymph capillaries.

3 How to Identify Lymphatic Capillaries

In the collapsed stage, with such attenuated endothelium and narrow lumina, the lymphatics would not be identified in routine histological preparations on hematoxylin and eosin sections. It is difficult or impossible to differentiate them from interstitial spaces and their closely apposed endothelial cells from connective tissue cells. The dilated lymphatics are difficult to differentiate from blood capillaries.

The lymphatics can be visualized by orcein or Weigert's staining (resorcin-fuchsin) due to the elastic fibers surrounding the capillaries (MORTIMER et al. 1983; OHKUMA 1982; PFLEGER 1964a). Blood capillaries do not possess any elastic fibers unless they are large enough to have an internal elastic lamina (Fig. 1). GOMORI's method demonstrates the argyrophil microfilaments (Fig. 2) surrounding the lymphatic capillary (PFLEGER 1964a).

For electron-microscopic studies, resin-embedded semithin sections stained with toluidine blue are much more suitable for revealing the lymphatics than the much thicker paraffin-embedded specimens. This level of resolution is good enough to establish the existence of lymphatic vessels but not good enough to distinguish the main morphological features of the capillaries.

The dermal lymphatics have been studied by various authors in biopsy material from different species and from different regions of the body. They found that it was possible to discuss the electron-microscopic morphology of the mammalian dermal lymphatics in general, at least of those species that have been studied up to the present time.

Lymphatic capillaries possess specific morphological features that differentiate them from the dermal blood capillaries:

1. The lumen is irregular in shape.
2. The endothelium is extremely attenuated.
3. The perivascular basal lamina is discontinuous.
4. Interendothelial gaps are common.
5. Pericytes are missing.
6. The lymphatic capillary is surrounded by elastic fibers, but a continuous elastic lamina is lacking (Figs. 3, 4).
7. Specific microfilaments terminate on the abluminal membrane of the capillary endothelial cells.

Enzyme histochemical methods may also help to differentiate the cutaneous lymphatics from blood capillaries. Aminopeptidase and acid-*p*-nitrophenyl phosphatase reactions proved to be negative for lymphatics, while the blood capillaries displayed positivity in the wall (NISHIDA and OHKUMA 1983).

The normal lymphatic endothelium lacked the enzymes alkaline phosphatase and ATP-ase but showed strong 5'-nucleotidase reaction. The normal blood capillary endothelium was positive for the enzymes alkaline phosphatase, 5'-nucleotidase, and ATP-ase (OHKUMA 1982).

The *immunohistochemical methods* have provided new possibilities for distinguishing lymphatics from blood vessels.

There is agreement on the localization of factor VIII-related antigen (F VIIIRA) in blood endothelial cells but opinions are not unanimous concerning the demonstration of F VIIIRA in the endothelial cells of lymphatics because of the difficulty in documenting lymphatics. MUKAI et al. (1980) found a negative reaction for F VIIIRA in normal lymphatic vessels and the sinuses of lymph nodes.

In recent years F VIIIRA positivity has been documented in the lymphatic endothelial cells, but the most intensive reactions were produced in cryostat sections. The intensity of the reactions was weak and patchy when compared with the endothelium of blood vessels (BECK-STEAD et al. 1985; SVANHOLM et al. 1984). The results of these studies suggest that the lymphatic endothelium might produce this antigen in very small amounts (BECKSTEAD et al. 1985).

Monoclonal antibodies (PAL-E) markedly stain the endothelium of blood capillaries and small veins in human frozen sections but do not stain lymphatic endothelium (SCHLINGEMANN et al. 1985).

A continuous basal lamina is lacking around the dermal lymphatic capillaries. The elastic and collagen fibers are directly connected with the capillary endothelium (Fig. 5).

The shape of the lumen is variable. Collapsed lymphatic capillaries have a split lumen and sometimes it is difficult to distinguish them from connective tissue cells (Figs. 6–8). The shape of the dilated lumen is irregular (Figs. 5, 10, 13, 14). Five main types of interendothelial connections have been observed (LEAK 1971; YANG et al. 1981): end-to-end connections, interdigitating, overlapping, tight, and desmosome-like junctions. The variability of these interendothelial junctions is great. The end-to-end connection is rare. Most probably it represents a temporary connection between the tips of the elongated endothelial cell processes (see Fig. 126). The convoluted, undulating cell processes can form very complicated interdigitations (Figs. 5, 7–9).

The overlapping connection is the most characteristic intercellular contact between lymphatic capillary endothelial cells. The overlapping cell processes are demonstrable also on scanning electron-microscopic pictures (CASTENHOLZ 1986). The elongated endothelial processes can overlap each other without displaying intermembranous junctions (Figs. 7, 8). Desmosomal junctions (Fig. 9) and tight junctions (Figs. 11, 12) are also observed between the cellular membranes of the multiple overlapping endothelial processes.

The extremely irregular shape of the lymphatic capillaries may result in complicated configurations on section planes (Fig. 13). The infolded and undulated endothelial cell loops can produce unusual lumen variations (Figs. 14, 15) and accordion-like wrinkling of the wall (Figs. 16, 17).

Fig. 1. Lymphedema, human lower leg, skin. Venules (V), arterioles (A) and lymphatic capillaries (L) are seen in the dermis. The lymphatic vessels contain erythrocytes and they are surrounded by elastic fibers. Orcein, × 150

Fig. 2. Normal human skin, forearm. The argyrophil microfilaments around the dermal lymphatic capillary (arrow) border the lymphatic lumen. Gomori's stain, × 120

Fig. 3. Normal human skin, forearm. The elastic fibers are missing (arrows) along some portions of the lymphatic wall. Orcein, × 150

Fig. 4. The same dermal lymphatic as in Fig. 3, but another section is demonstrated from the series. The elastic fibers are running parallel to the long axis of the vessel and they are missing along a short segment of the wall (arrow). Orcein, × 150

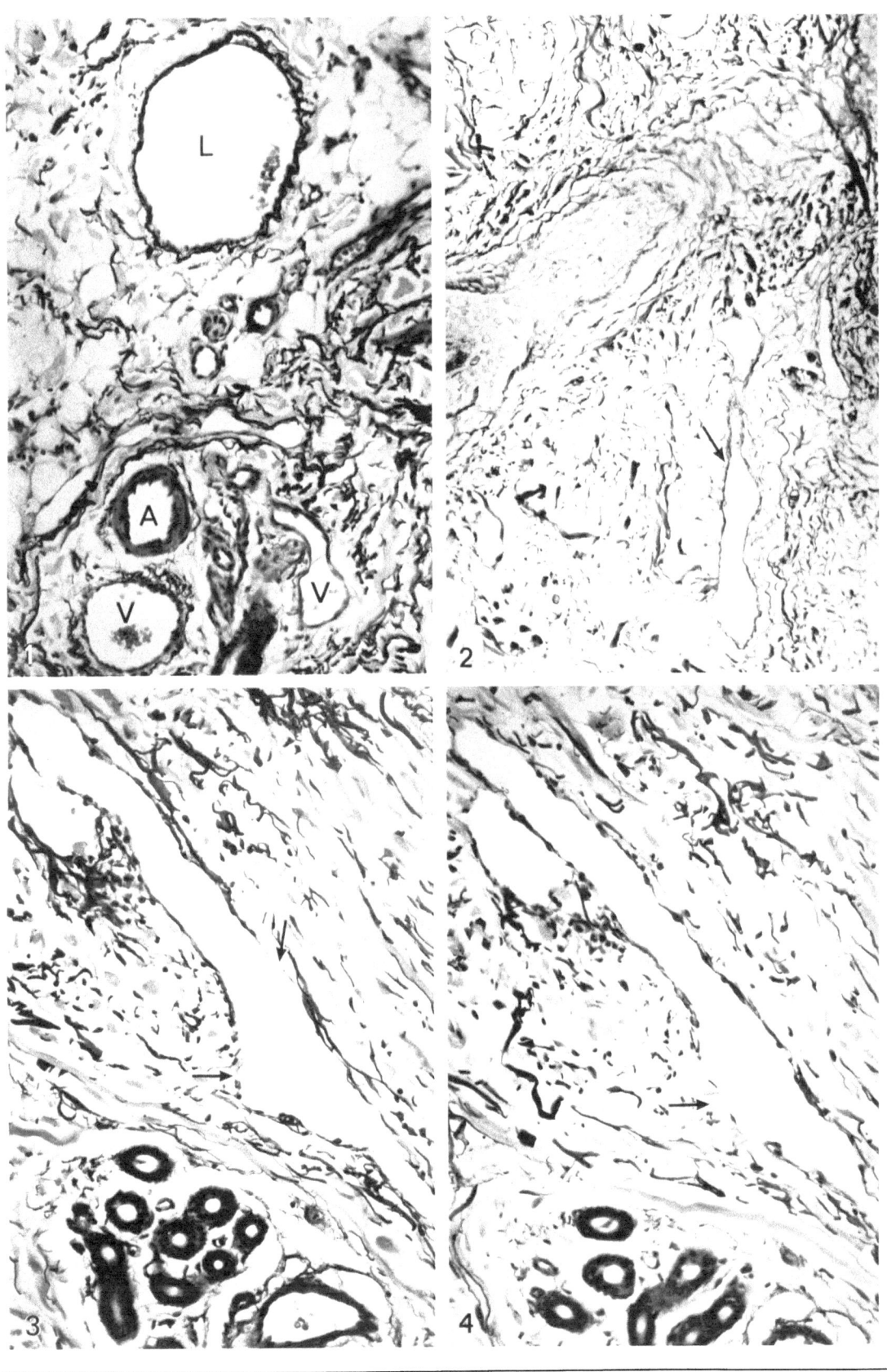

Fig. 5. Normal human skin, lower leg. The basal lamina is missing. A patent junction is seen *(star)* between the endothelial processes. The endothelial cells are connected by junctions *(arrow)* or they are interdigitating *(double arrow).* The cytoplasm is rich in organelles. × 2000

Fig. 6. Normal skin, rat paw. The lumen is very narrow. The basal lamina *(Bl)* is discontinuous. The overlapping endothelial cell processes are connected by junctions or interdigitating. The connective tissue microfilaments are numerous around the lymphatic capillary. × 5000

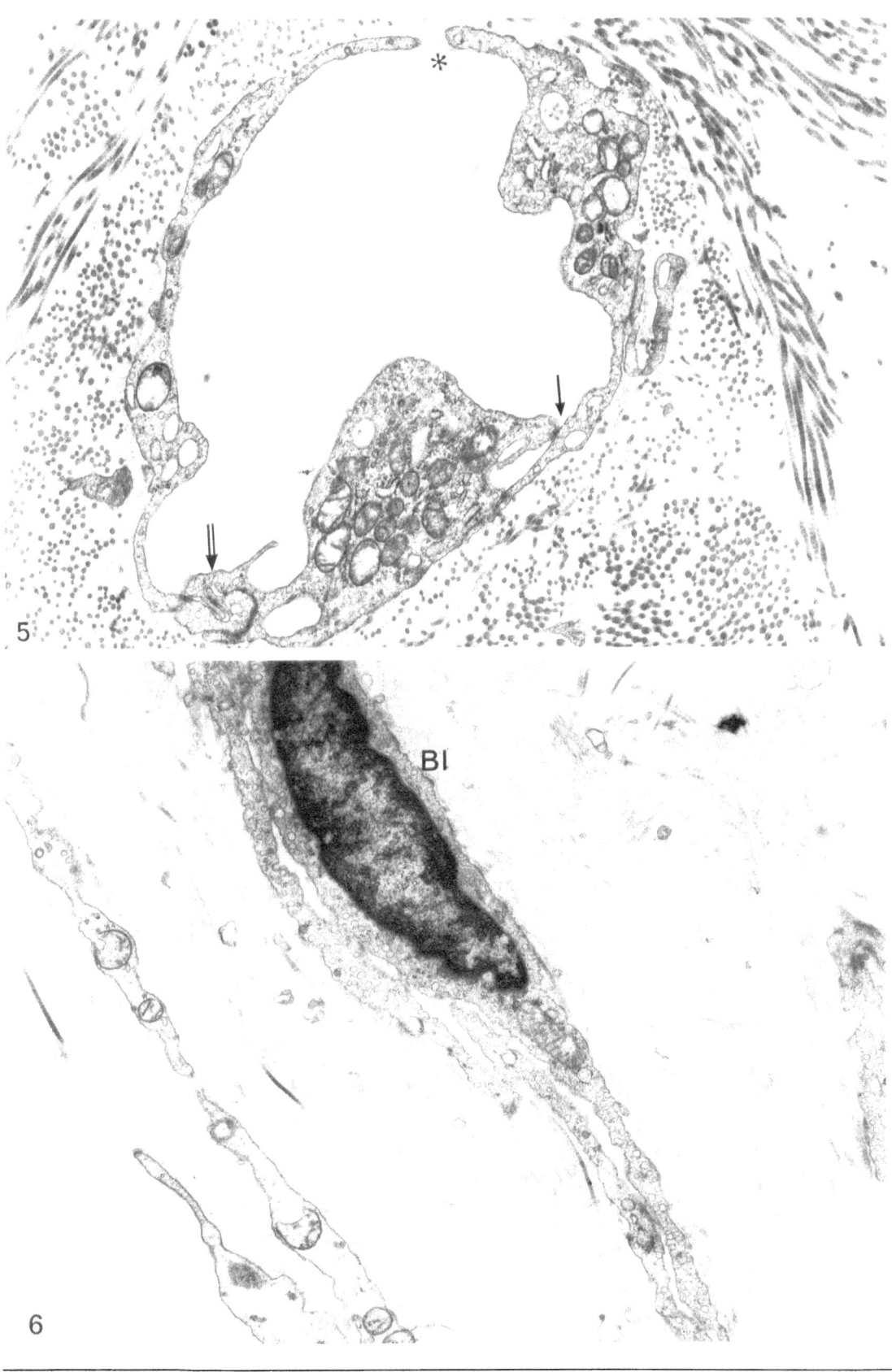

Fig. 7. Human skin, hyperkeratosis, lower leg. The thin convoluted, undulating endothelial processes overlap each other. The basal lamina is missing. The collagen fibers *(Co)* and the connective tissue microfilaments are directly connected with the capillary wall. × 4000

Fig. 8. Human skin, hyperkeratosis, back. Only a split lumen is seen between the overlapping thin endothelial processes *(star)*. In the vicinity of the necklike isthmus of the lymphatic capillary the lumen *(Lu)* is expanded. This portion of the wall protrudes into the connective tissue like a spike. A cotton-like coat of microfilaments is seen around the capillary. × 5400

Fig. 9. Human skin, hyperkeratosis, back. The thin endothelial cell processes of the lymphatic capillary are interdigitated and overlap each other. Desmosome-like junctions are seen between the overlapping endothelial processes. The basal lamina is missing; the collagen fibers are in direct contact with the endothelial membrane. processes. The basal lamina is missing; the collagen fibers are in direct contact with the endothelial membrane. × 12500

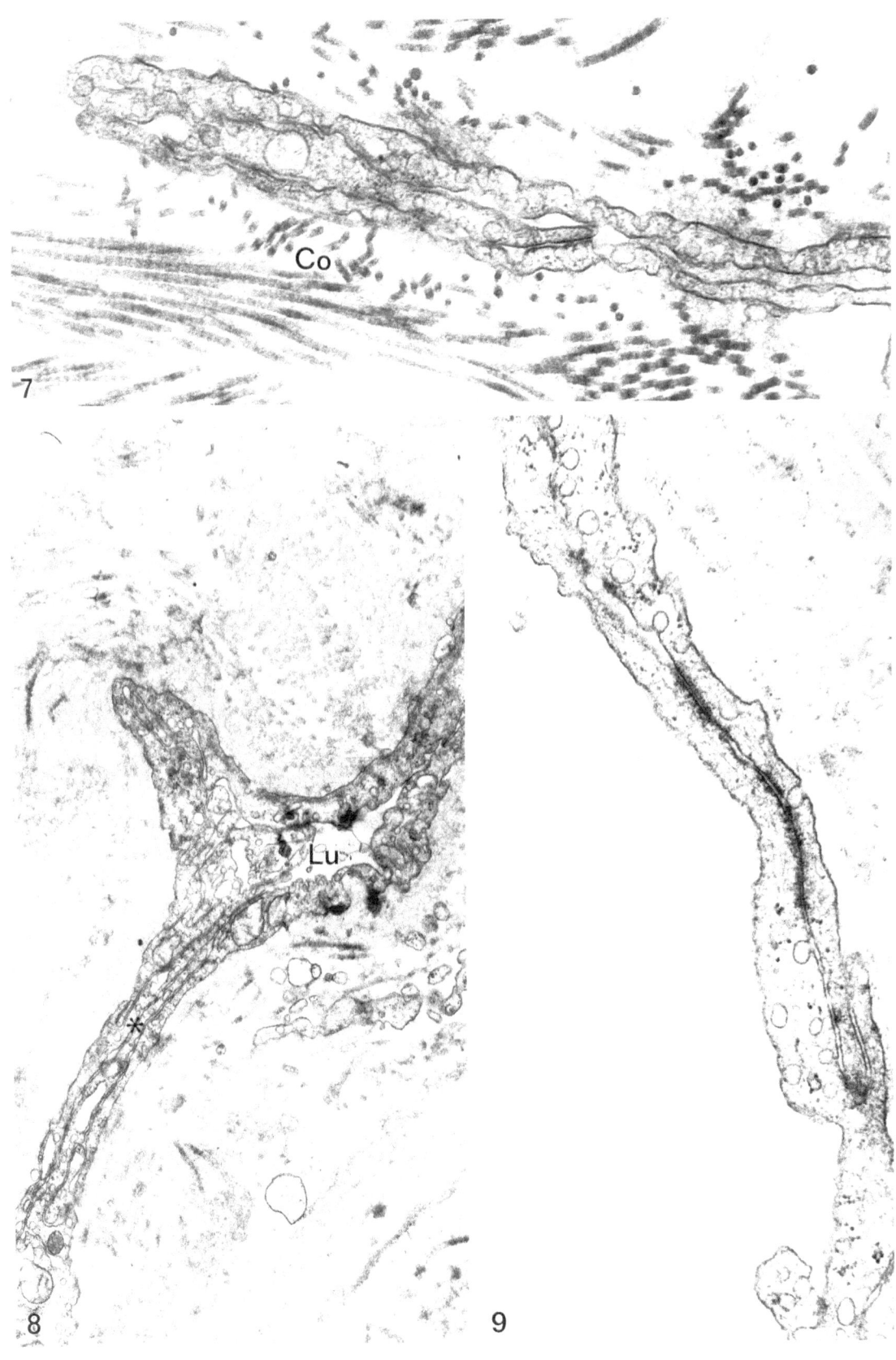

Fig. 10. Normal skin, rat paw. The accordion-like infoldings of the thin endothelial processes border the dilated lumen *(Lu)*. The cytoplasm has numerous vacuoles. The connective tissue filaments and the collagen fibers surround the lymphatic capillary. × 12000

Fig. 11. Normal skin, rat paw. The multiple overlapping flat endothelial cell processes are rich in pinocytotic vesicles. Between two overlapping processes tight junctions are present *(arrows)*. The basal lamina is missing. The connective tissue filaments are connected directly with the abluminal cell membrane of the endothelial cell. × 14000

Fig. 12. Normal skin, rat paw. The overlapping cytoplasmic processes of the endothelial cells contain numerous organelles. Dense plates represent the intermembranous junctions *(arrow)*. The basal lamina *(Bl)* is discontinuous. The connective tissue microfilaments run directly to the cell membrane of the endothelial cells. × 10000

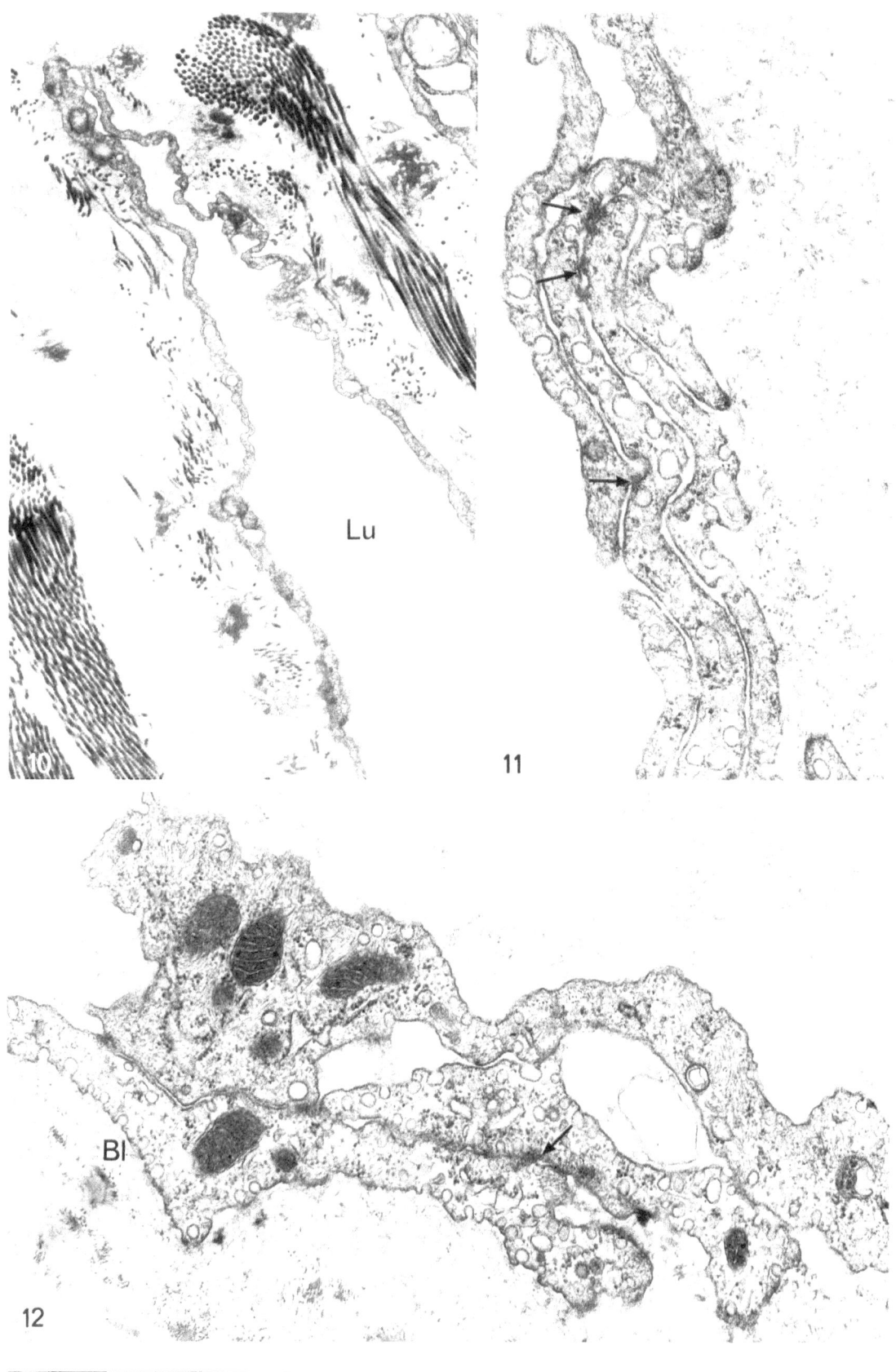

Fig. 13. Normal skin, canine hind limb. There are five lumina *(Lu$_{1-5}$)* of varying shape and dilatation stage. The endothelial cells are mainly flat, but some cells possess indented nuclei and these cells bulge into the lumen. × 2000

Fig. 14. Normal skin, canine hind limb. A complicated channel system is developed by the bizarre wrinkling of the flat endothelial cells. The elastic and collagen fibrils are connected with the abluminal membrane of the endothelial cells. It is probable that the three-dimensional channel system could be cut along the proposed line of section *(arrows)* to result in the multiple lumina complex of Fig. 13. × 5500

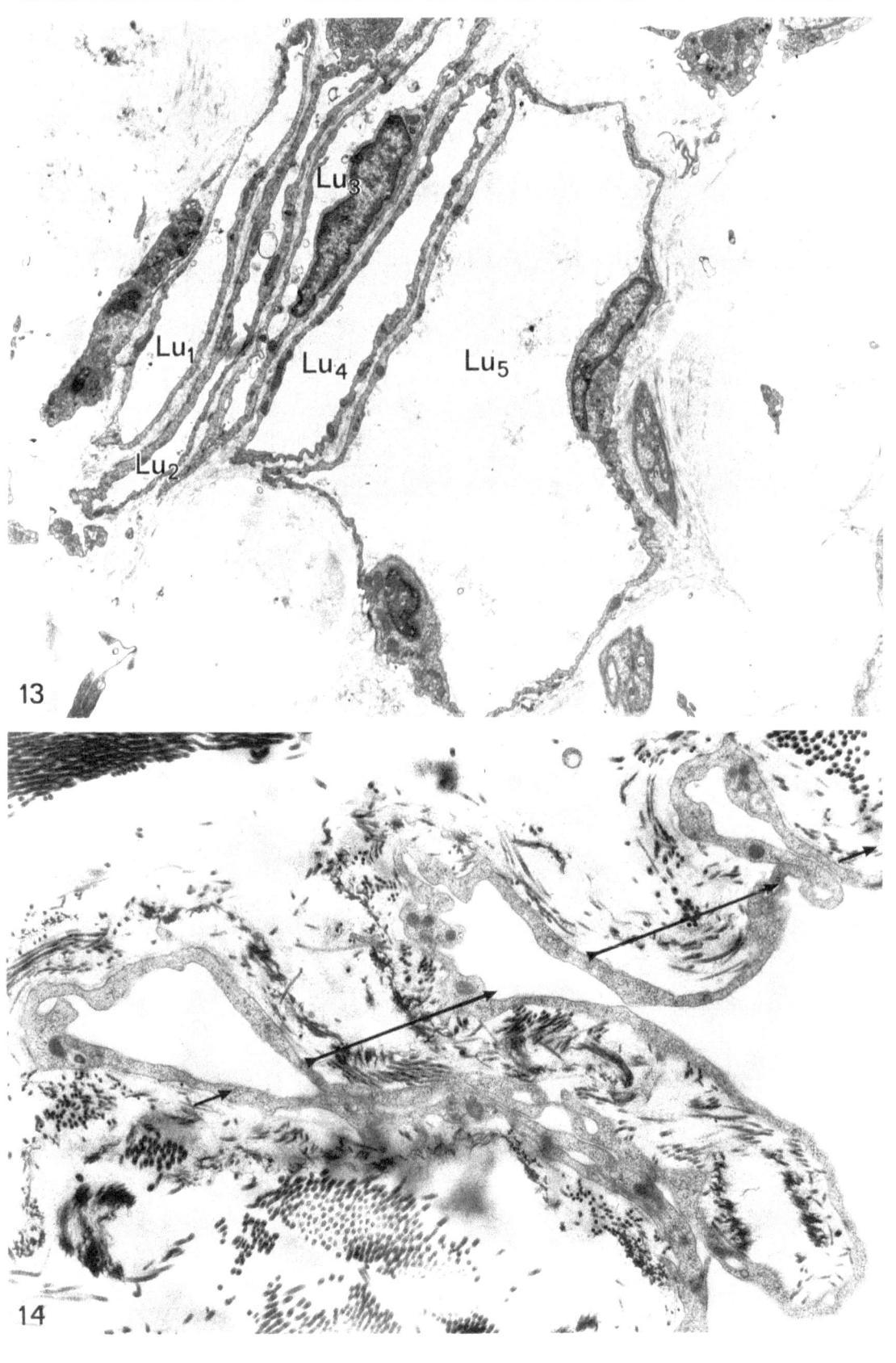

Fig. 15. Lymphedema, human lower leg. Folded endothelial cells form a loop with a nucleated endothelial cell on the tip *(End)*. This loop bulges into the lumen *(Lu)*. The prelymphatic space *(star)* is filled with a fine granular substance. × 5000

Fig. 16. Normal skin, canine hind limb. The endothelial loop protrudes into the lumen. The membranes of the folded endothelial cell are closely attached. The basal lamina is missing. × 19000

Fig. 17. Normal skin, canine hind limb. The accordion-like feature of the lymphatic wall develops due to the folding of the endothelial cell. The connective tissue fibers are directly connected with the endothelial membrane. × 14000

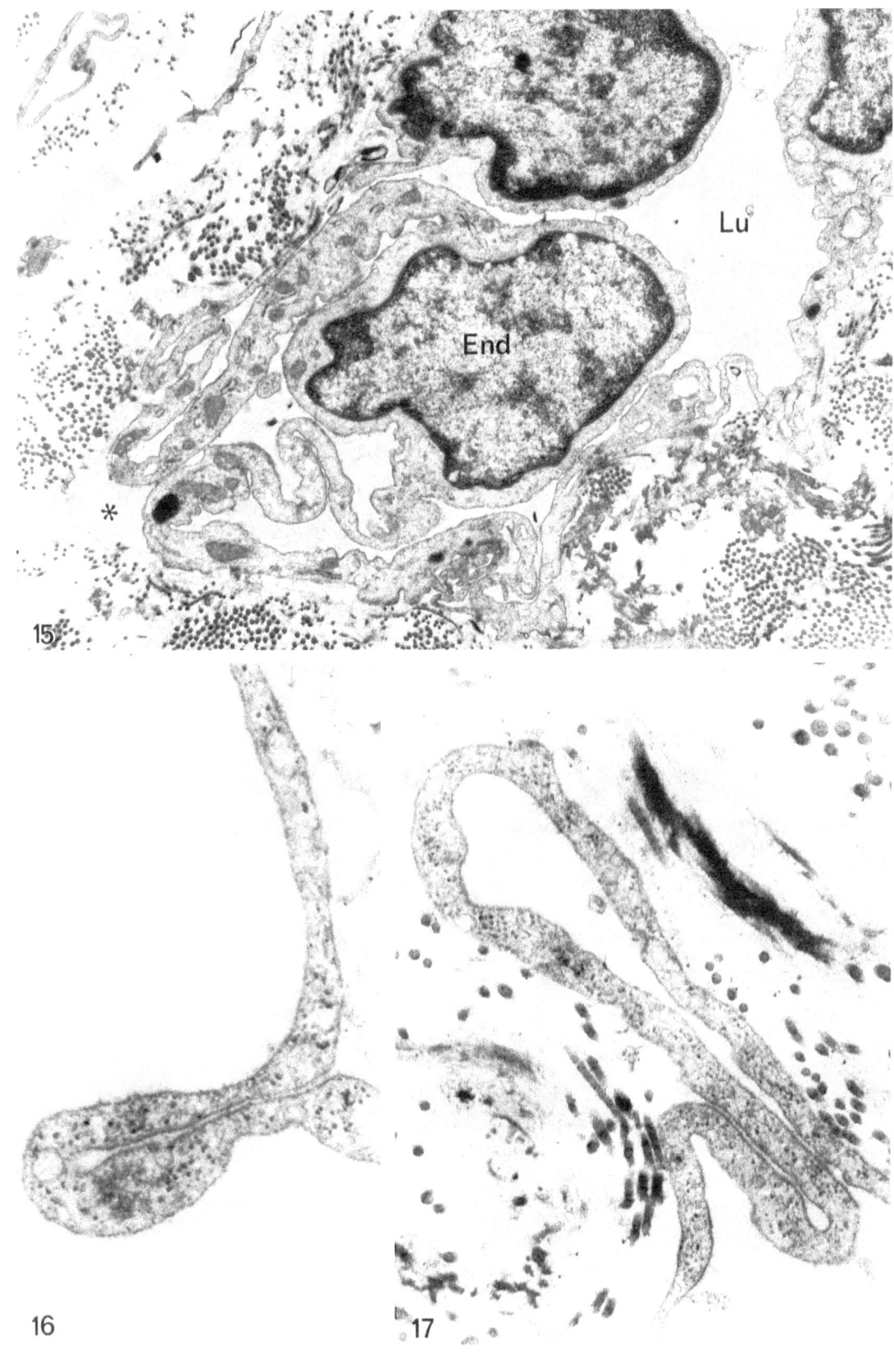

4 Morphological Features of the Dermal Lymphatic Capillary

4.1 Pericapillary Connective Tissue

The abluminal endothelial surface of the dermal lymphatic capillaries has special contacts with the pericapillary connective tissue.

4.1.1 Basal Lamina

A continuous basal lamina is lacking. The discontinuous basal lamina consists of very fine filaments embedded in a loose matrix. The thickness of the basal lamina is very variable; sometimes it can be multiplied. Its arrangement is irregular and the basal lamina escorting the dense cytoplasmic plates can be very prominent (Figs. 18 and 26). The basal lamina is missing along the dense cytoplasmic plates where the elastic microtubuli and connective tissue microfilaments are attached to the endothelial cytoplasm (Figs. 21–23).

4.1.2 Endothelial Cytoplasmic Pseudopodia

The numerous cytoplasmic pseudopodia protruding into the surrounding interstitium can produce a complicated joining surface between the lymphatic endothelium and the perivascular connective tissue (Fig. 18). The cytoplasmic "spines" may be connected with specific perilymphatic connective tissue microfilaments (Figs. 19, 20, 23).

4.1.3 Connective Tissue Microfilaments

LEAK and BURKE (1968) presented filaments in close association with the lymphatic wall. Two classes of filaments are recognized in close contact with the abluminal endothelial surface: Filaments with diameters of 10–12 nm vary in length. In cross sections they have light cores surrounded by a dense outer layer, suggesting a different affinity of the medulla and cortex for osmium-uranyl-lead stains used to contrast the ultrathin sections. The filaments exhibit an irregular beaded pattern along their long axis. The longitudinal periodicity measures 10–12 nm. To summarize: the filaments have hollow profiles imitating tubules; they measure 10–12 nm in diameter; their length varies; their longitudinal periodicity is irregular, measuring about 9–12 nm. They are not densely stained with phosphotungstic acid as are elastic fibers.

The microfilaments were supposed to be identical with elastic microtubules (LEAK and BURKE 1968). The outer leaflet of the endothelial cell membrane, stained with ruthenium red (a dye that is binding to the mucopolysaccharide component of the external membrane coat), demonstrated a thick, fuzzy coat in which the microfilaments seemed to be inserted (LEAK 1972a).

Sometimes the tubular microfilaments are observed to be arranged in bundles running parallel with the endothelial membranes (Fig. 24). These filaments connect the endothelial cells directly to the surrounding interstitium. The term "lymphatic anchoring filaments" was used to describe the function and the intimate contact between lymphatic endothelium and filaments. However, there are four reasons why we prefer the term "lymphatic elastic microtubules". They are as follows:

1. The filaments possess the same morphological features as those of elastic microfilaments (hollow profile, beaded pattern, same diameter).
2. The elastic microtubules running directly to the abluminal endothelial cell membrane are connected with elastic matrix. The elastic fibers anchor the lymphatic endothelium to the pericapillary interstitium (Figs. 19 and 23).
3. The term "anchoring filament" can be misleading because the same technical term is used to characterize the function of the microfilaments connecting the epidermal junctional zone to the connective tissue.
4. Along the lymphatic endothelium another filamentous network exists, consisting of filaments of 4–6 nm in diameter. These filaments are also anchored to the abluminal surface of the capillary endothelial cells and are connected with the adjoining connective tissue. They were described by LEAK and BURKE (1968).

Filaments of 4–6 nm in diameter form a network between the abluminal endothelial surface of the lymphatic capillary and the adjoining connective tissue components. The bundles of the filaments are arranged parallel to the long axis of the lymphatic capillary wall. These filaments can be connected with the dense cytoplasmic plates situated along the abluminal endothelial surface (Fig. 25). They are intermingled with the perivascular collagen fibers and are called "fine" or "connective tissue" microfilaments.

4.1.4 Attachment Plates Along the Capillary Wall

There are two different types of attachment plates along the abluminal surface of the capillary endothelium. They can be distinguished on the basis of their substructure, and they serve as attachment plates for connective tissue microfilaments.

Hemidesmosome-like cytoplasmic plates are associated with cytoplasmic microfilaments, 6–8 nm in diameter, running to the dense cytoplasmic plate. The lymphatic elastic microtubules are attached in higher numbers to the desmosome-like cytoplasmic plates than they are along the interdesmosomal endothelial segments (Figs. 20, 21, 23).

The second type of dense plate consists of actin-like microfilaments measuring 4–6 nm in diameter, running parallel with the abluminal endothelial membrane (Figs. 24, 25).

4.1.5 Elastic Fibers

The dermal lymphatic capillaries are surrounded by elastic fibers. The histological demonstration of the elastic network around the capillaries (by orcein) is acceptable for identifing dermal lymphatic capillaries (MORTIMER et al.; OHKUMA 1982; PFLEGER 1964). The elastic fibers do not form a continuous elastic lamina around the capillaries (Figs. 3, 4, 27–30).

The elastic fibers can be directly connected with the abluminal endothelial membrane (Figs. 19, 23); they are observed in close vicinity to the capillary endothelium (Fig. 29), and they can be revealed in the perivascular space apart from the endothelium (Figs. 28, 31).

The elastic fibers may be oriented parallel with the long axis of the capillary lumen (Fig. 20), and they may be demonstrated running vertical to the endothelial membrane (Figs. 23, 55).

There are long segments of the lymphatic capillaries where the elastic fibers may be very prominent, but there are other segments where the elastic fibers are missing from the perivascular interstitium or appear spotty along the capillary wall (Figs. 30, 32). It is suggested that the dermal lymphatic capillary is surrounded by elastic fibers arranged in a spiral pattern (Fig. 33). The spiral pattern of the elastic fibers can explain the controversy over interpreting the presence of the pericapillary elastic coat (see Schema 1).

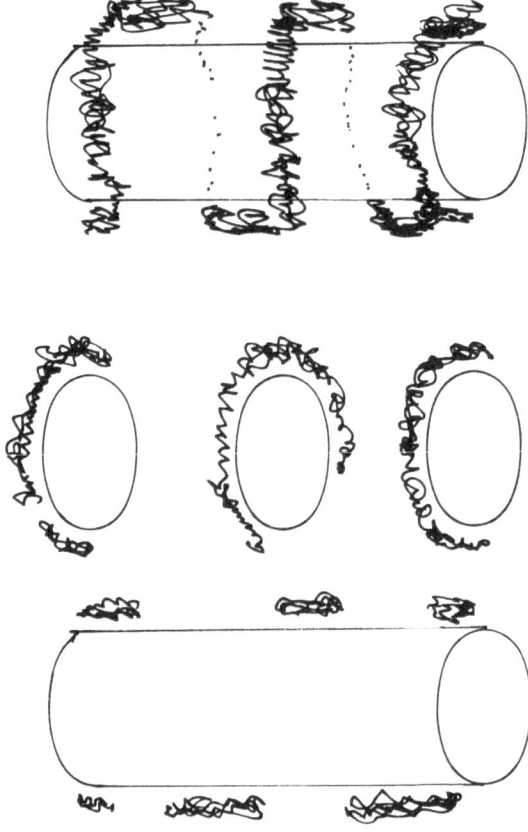

Schema 1. The schema shows the suggested arrangement of the elastic fibers around the lymphatic capillary. The elastic spire appears in different patterns on the cross and longitudinal sections

4.1.6 Collagen Fibers

PULLINGER and FLOREY (1935) observed collagen fibers in close proximity to the lymphatic endothelium. CASLEY-SMITH and FLOREY (1961) described bundles of collagen running to the lymphatic capillaries.

Collagen fibers are embedded in the granulofilamentous ground substance of the pericapillary space. Occasionally their contacts with the lymphatic endothelium can be demonstrated (Figs. 26, 46).

4.2 Endothelial Cells

Endothelial cells line the inside of lymphatic capillaries. These cells play an important role in permeability and transport function and in mediating their response to different pathological and pathophysiological stimuli. The ultrastructural morphology of the lymphatic endothelial cells has been reviewed by LEAK (1976). The general organization of the lymphatic capillary endothelium follows.

4.2.1 Cytoplasmic Microfilaments

The microfilament content of the endothelial cells varies according to the activity of the portion of the capillary studied. In cases of special activity the modified endothelial cell can be full of microfilaments 6–7 nm in diameter (Fig. 34). The existence of the microfilaments is not always obvious on the section planes because of their very fine measurements on cross sections (Fig. 35).

a. *Microfilaments of 6–7 nm in diameter* can display an irregular longitudinal periodicity measuring approximately 10 nm (Fig. 36). This type of filament is seen in lymphatics without a smooth muscle cell layer (SCHIPP 1968).

The filaments are dispersed in the cytoplasm, but (a) in some places they may aggregate, forming desmosome-like plates along the abluminal surface of the capillary endothelium (Figs. 18, 21), or (b) they may be arranged in bundles (Fig. 36). The intermediate-sized filaments proved to be vimentin.

b. *Microfilaments of 4–6 nm in diameter* are also dispersed in the cytoplasm but (a) they may be aggregated around the nuclei (Fig. 35) or (b) they may be arranged in bundles, forming dense plates along the abluminal cell membrane of the capillary endothelial cells (Figs. 24 and 25). The smaller microfilaments are supposed to be actin-like filaments.

4.2.2 Microtubules

Microtubules measuring approximately 25 nm in diameter occur in close association with centrioles, but they are frequently demonstrated throughout other cytoplasmic areas as well (Figs. 20 and 21).

4.2.3 Multivesicular Bodies

The appearance of large cytoplasmic vacuole-containing vesicles measuring 20–40 nm in diameter and limited to the membrane is not common (Fig. 37). They are not identical with the multitubular endothelial bodies as suggested by POGGI et al. (1986). The tubular cytoplasmic rods described by WEIBEL and PALADE (1964) have not yet been found in the endothelium of dermal lymphatic capillaries.

4.2.4 Golgi Apparatus

The Golgi apparatus may be well developed, showing dilated tubules and cisternae (Figs. 38, 40).

4.2.5 Centrioles

Centrioles or pairs of centrioles occur in the perinuclear region of the capillary endothelial cell (Fig. 38).

4.2.6 Mitochondria

Mitochondria are randomly distributed in the cytoplasm, but they may be concentrated in high numbers in the perinuclear regions or in other segments of the cytoplasm (Fig. 39).

4.2.7 Endoplasmic Reticulum

Endoplasmic reticulum is usually not prominent. Short segments of tubules and dilated cisternae are seen randomly scattered in the cytoplasm. The perinuclear endoplasmic reticulum may form unique tetramembranous complexes (Fig. 40).

4.2.8 Ribosomes

Many ribosomes are scattered throughout the cytoplasmic matrix. They appear in single units and also in clusters or as polyribosomes (Figs. 36, 40).

4.2.9 Cilia

Cilia with extracellular whips have been observed on rare occasions. Basal bodies of the cilia have been not infrequently seen in the central cytoplasm of the endothelial cells (Fig. 41).

4.2.10 Lipid Droplets

The number of endothelial lipid droplets is increased in lymphedema. The lipid droplets are partially membrane bound, surrounded by collapsed tubules of endoplasmic reticulum (Fig. 42). The macrophages and perilymphatic connective tissue cells are loaded with numerous lipid droplets varying in size and density (Fig. 43).

4.2.11 Vesicles

Several types of cytoplasmic vesicles occur in the endothelial cells. *Pinocytotic vesicles* measuring approximately 80–100 nm in diameter can be revealed along both the luminal and abluminal surfaces of the capillary endothelium (Figs. 44 and 45). *Cytoplasmic vesicles* of different sizes are found, 80–200 nm. *Coated vesicles* measure about 100 nm in diameter.

The pinocytotic vesicles have a considerable tendency to fuse. The vesicles may form chains due to the fusion of their membranes, and these chains seem to connect both the luminal and the abluminal spaces (Fig. 46). Since the existence of chains of vesicles formed by fusion in the endothelium of blood capillaries was described by PALADE and BRUNS (1968) and SIMI-

ONESCU et al. (1975), comparable channels have been suggested in lymphatic endothelium (JONES et al. 1983).

The cytoplasmic vesicles are supposed to be members of the transendothelial passageway, being transported across the endothelial cytoplasm.

The coated vesicles are usually seen along the abluminal surface of the capillary endothelium. The insertion of elastic microtubules by coated vesicles has been described without comment by LEAK and BURKE (1968). We have found this phenomen to be very rare and suggest that the filament attached closely to the membrane might be only temporarily inserted in the vesicle (Fig. 47). The insertion might be due to the active membrane changes along the lymphatic endothelium reacting with the directly connected connective tissue microfilaments.

Endothelial fenestrae like those seen in blood capillaries (ELFVIN 1965) have not been found in dermal lymphatic capillaries. Vesicles closed by a diaphragm showing a central dense knob were discovered along the luminal surface of the lymphatic capillary (Fig. 45), but the low incidence of vesicles with a diaphragm suggests that membrane fusion is a rapid process.

4.2.12 Lysosomes

In contrast to inflammatory conditions, lysosomes are rare in the normal lymphatic endothelium. The lysosomes contain different particles (Fig. 48).

4.2.13 Dense Granules

Dense granules of varying size have been observed in some endothelial cells; however, it was not possible to determine the substructure of the membrane-bound granules (Fig. 43).

4.2.14 Tubuloreticular and Crystalloid Inclusions

Tubuloreticular and crystalloid inclusions were found in human and animal lymphatic endothelial cells under both normal and various pathological conditions (Figs. 48–50). The tubuloreticular structure consists of reticular aggregates of membranous tubules measuring 25–28 nm in diameter, located within the cisternae of endoplasmic reticulum (Figs. 49, 50) and the perinuclear envelope (Fig. 42).

In human dermal lymphatic capillaries the tubuloreticular structures are composed of loose reticular aggregates of tubules. In animal tissues (ALBERTINE et al. 1980) they display a paracrystalline organization (Fig. 48). The tubuloreticular structures have been proven to be pathological variations of the endoplasmic reticulum (GRIMLEY and SCHAFF 1976).

4.2.15 Nucleus

The shape of the nucleus varies depending on the phase of endothelial contraction. In the dilated capillaries the nuclei are oval or rod-shaped with a smooth contour. In the contracted endothelial cells the nuclei appear to be irregular in shape and deeply indented. Nuclear blebs are not unusual (Fig. 51). Nucleoli are often revealed in the nucleoplasm, and nuclear bodies are also frequently observed (Figs. 51 and 52). Nuclear pseudoinclusions appear, due to the deep nuclear invaginations. On sections the cytoplasmic contents seem to be situated within the nucleoplasm (Fig. 52). The unique owl-eye nuclear inclusion is assumed to be a remnant of lipid droplets (Fig. 53).

4.3 Innervation

The lymphatic capillaries do not have any efferent nerve supply (silver impregnation in the mesentery) but they are in close attachment to sensory nerve endings (VAJDA 1966).

Closely surrounding and adjacent to the mesenteric lymphatics sensory endings of the Vater-Pacinian type were found (KUBIK and SZABÓ 1955).

The contractions of the larger lymphatic vessels, having smooth muscle cells in their adventitia, are modified by adrenergic and cholinergic nervous fibers and humoral factors.

Fig. 18. Inflammation, human skin, forearm. The endothelial cells containing large amounts of cytoplasmic microfilaments bulge into the lumen *(Lu)* and the cytoplasmic pseudopodia of the endothelial cells *(p)* protrude into the connective tissue surrounding the lymphatic capillary. × 5500

Fig. 19. Inflammation, eczematous rat paw skin. The spinelike cytoplasmic process of the lymphatic endothelial cell that protrudes into the connective tissue is directly connected with the microfilaments *(arrow)* of the elastic fiber *(E)*. There are some dense plates *(stars)* along the abluminal cell membrane of the endothelial cell. *NL*, Lymphatic lumen; × 22000

Fig. 20. Inflammation, eczematous rat paw skin. The shape of the lymphatic lumen *(Lu)* is irregular. The cytoplasm of the endothelial cells contains vesicles and microtubuli *(star)*. The thornlike cytoplasmic pseudopodium invades deep into the perivascular space. The connective tissue microfilaments are anchored directly to the cytoplasmic membrane and to the cytoplasmic dense plates *(arrows)*. × 10000

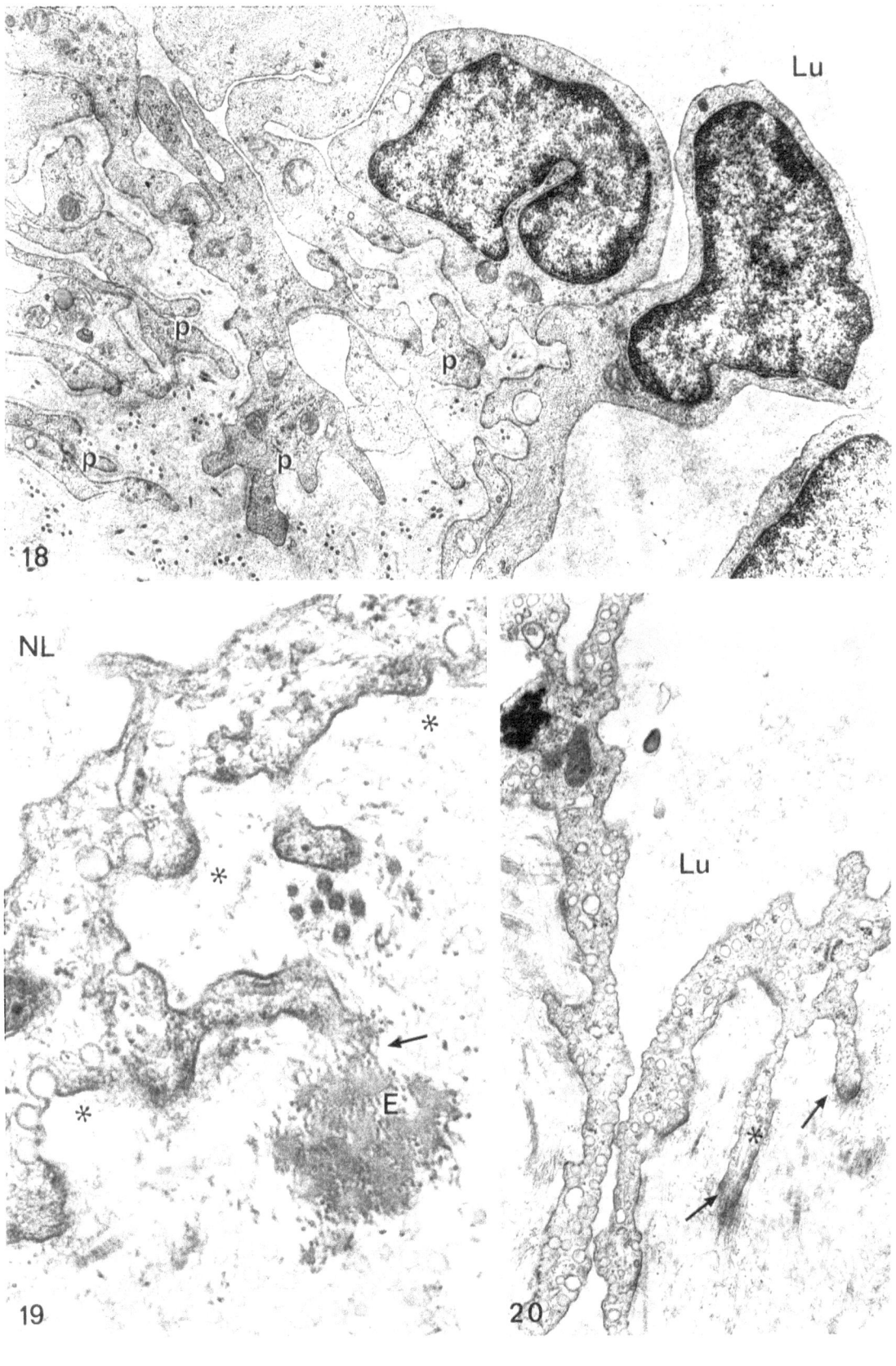

Fig. 21. Inflammation, rat paw skin. Numerous vesicles *(v)* and microtubules *(mt)* are seen in the cytoplasm of the lymphatic capillary endothelial cell. The basal lamina is missing. The tubular microfilaments *(f)* run directly to the abluminal cytoplasmic membrane. *Lu,* Lymphatic lumen; × 24000

Fig. 22. Inflammation, eczematous rat paw skin. The endothelial cytoplasm of the dilated lymphatic capillary is very rich in vesicles and vacuoles. The anchoring connective-tissue filaments run directly to the endothelial cell membrane and to the dense plates *(arrows)* along the abluminal cell membrane. *Lu,* Lymphatic lumen; × 8500

Fig. 23. Inflammation, eczematous rat paw skin. The basal lamina is missing around the lymphatic capillary. The anchoring connective-tissue filaments and the microfilaments of the elastic fiber *(E)* are connected directly with the dense plates *(arrows)* and with the abluminal membrane of the endothelial cells. *Lu,* Lymphatic lumen; × 9000

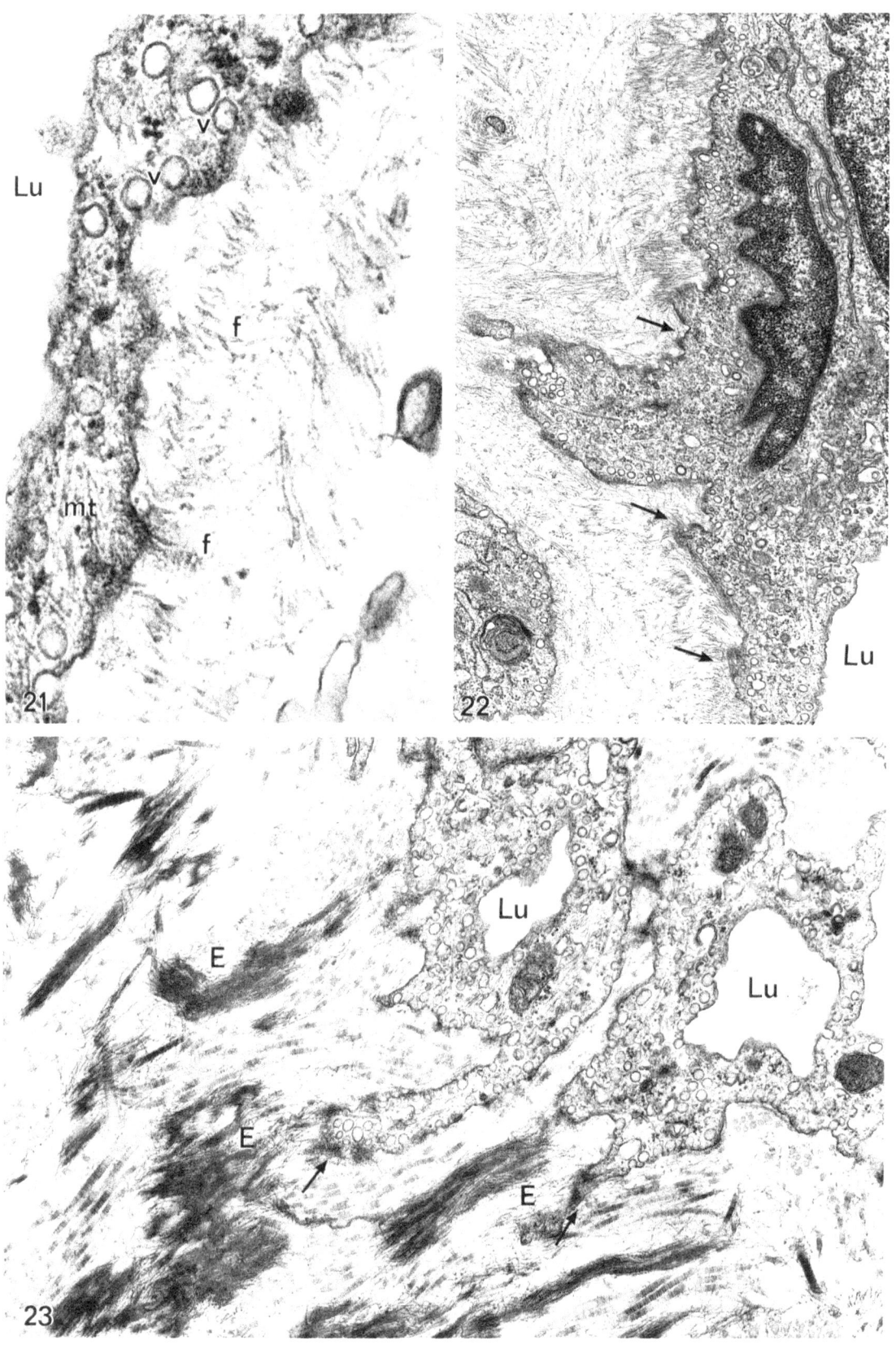

Fig. 24. Normal skin, rat paw. The cytoplasm of the endothelial cell is vacuolated. The dense plates *(stars)* of actin-like filaments along the peripheral cytoplasm are escorted by basal lamina fragments and parallel-running microfilaments showing longitudinal periodicity *(f)*. *Lu,* Lymphatic lumen; × 18000

Fig. 25. Lymphedema, human lower leg. The dilated lymphatic capillary is surrounded by a loose network of connective-tissue microfilaments. These filaments separate the capillary from the collagen fibers *(Co)*. The long peripheral dense plate *(arrow)* represents a bundle of parallelly arranged actin-like filaments. *Lu,* Lymphatic lumen; × 19500

Fig. 26. Inflammation, eczematous rat paw skin. The endothelial cell surrounding the lymphatic capillary lumen *(Lu)* contains pinocytotic vesicles. Along the dense cytoplasmic plates segments of basal lamina *(stars)* are seen. The collagen fibers *(Co)* are in close contact with the endothelial cell. × 20000

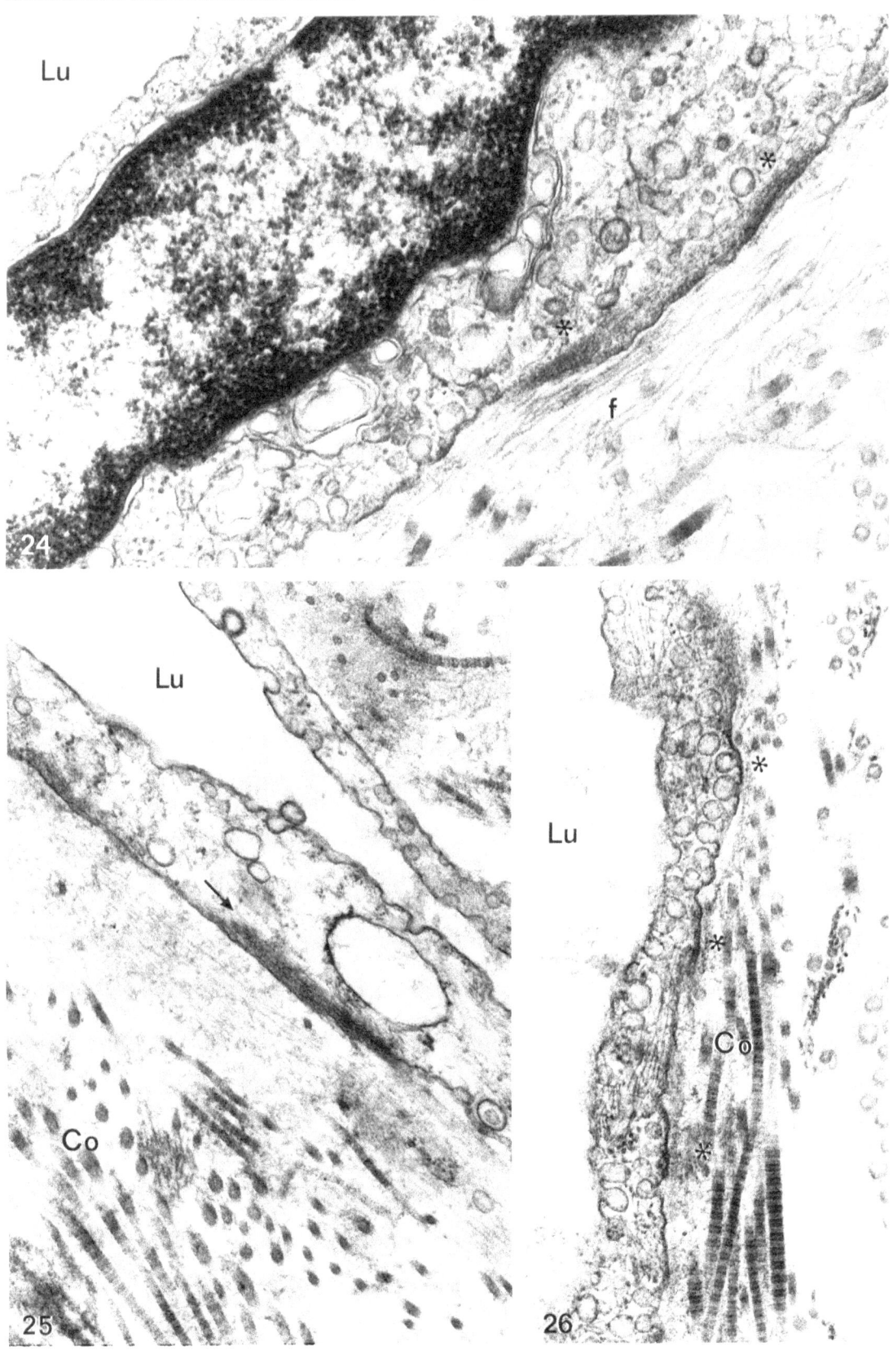

Fig. 27. Lymphedema, human lower leg. The dilated dermal lymphatic capillary is surrounded by elastic fibers. Toluidine blue, × 800

Fig. 28. Electron-microscopical picture of the dermal lymphatic capillary in Fig. 27. The elastic fibers *(E)* do not form a continuous elastic lamina. *Lu,* Lymphatic lumen; × 1500

Fig. 29. Normal skin, dog hind limb. The dermal lymphatic lumen is dilated *(Lu).* The attenuated endothelial cells are not surrounded by basal lamina. The lymphatic wall is directly connected with collagen fibers *(Co)* and with the microfilaments of the patchy cross sections of elastic fibers *(E).* × 8100

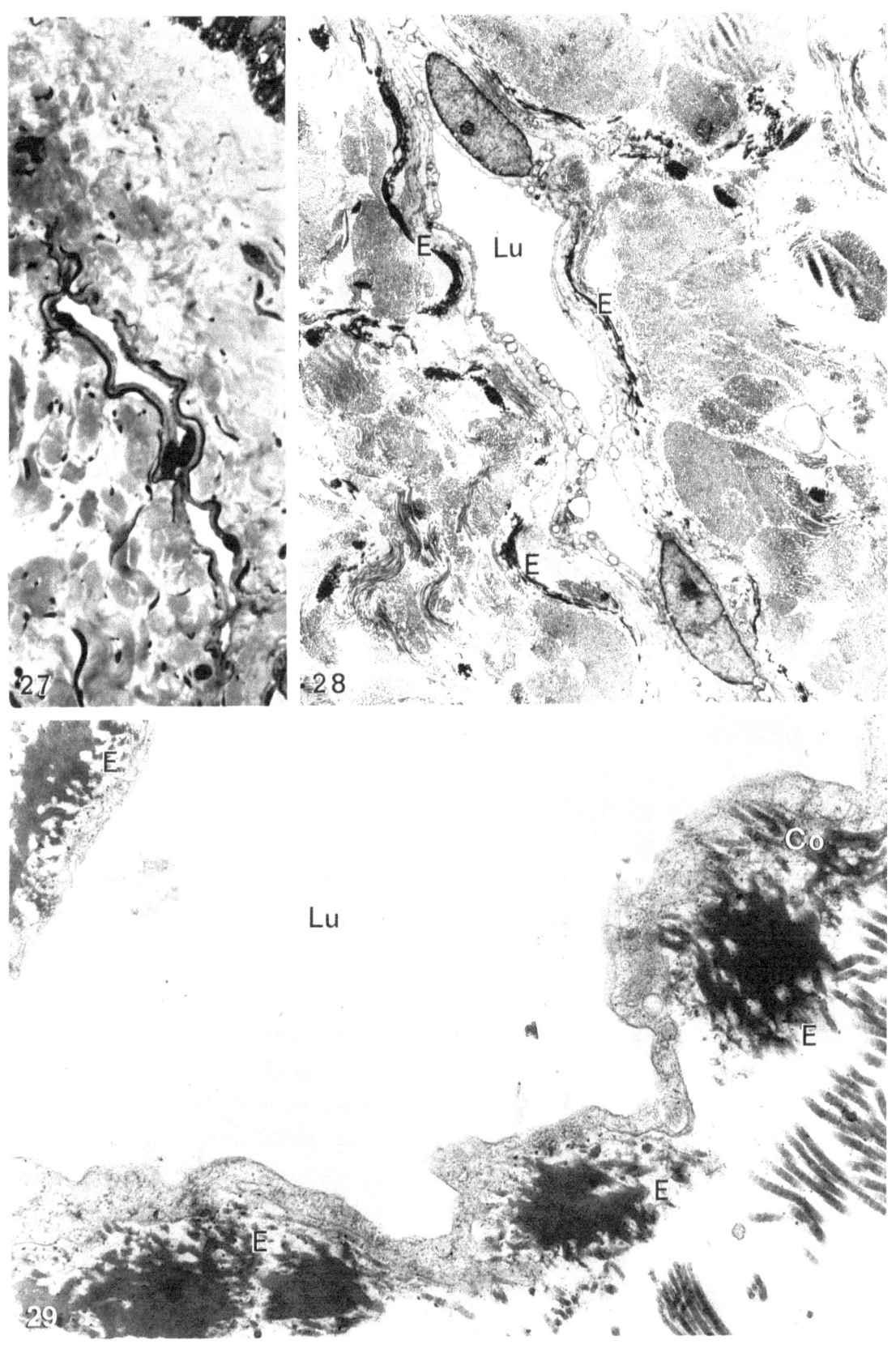

Fig. 30. Normal skin, canine hind limb.
a On the longitudinal section of the lympahtic capillary there are long portions *(stars)* where the capillary wall is surrounded by collagen fibers *(Co)* and the elastic fibers are missing.
b Elastic fibers *(E)* appear spotty along the lymphatic wall. *Lu,* Lymphatic lumen; × 8100

Fig. 31. Normal skin, canine hind limb. This portion of the lymphatic capillary is accompanied by elastic fibers *(E)* that do not have a direct connection with the endothelial membrane but accompany the lymphatic vessel in the "second row" of the perilymphatic interstitium. *Co,* Collagen fiber; *Ln,* lymphatic capillary; × 4800

Fig. 32. Normal skin, canine hind limb. The elastic fibers are missing in the perilymphatic space. The "naked" endothelial wall of the lymphatic capillary is surrounded by connective-tissue ground substance and collagen fibers. × 6400

Fig. 33. Due to the spiral arrangement of the elastic network, both cross and longitudinal sections of the elastic fibers are seen around the lymphatic capillary. × 8100

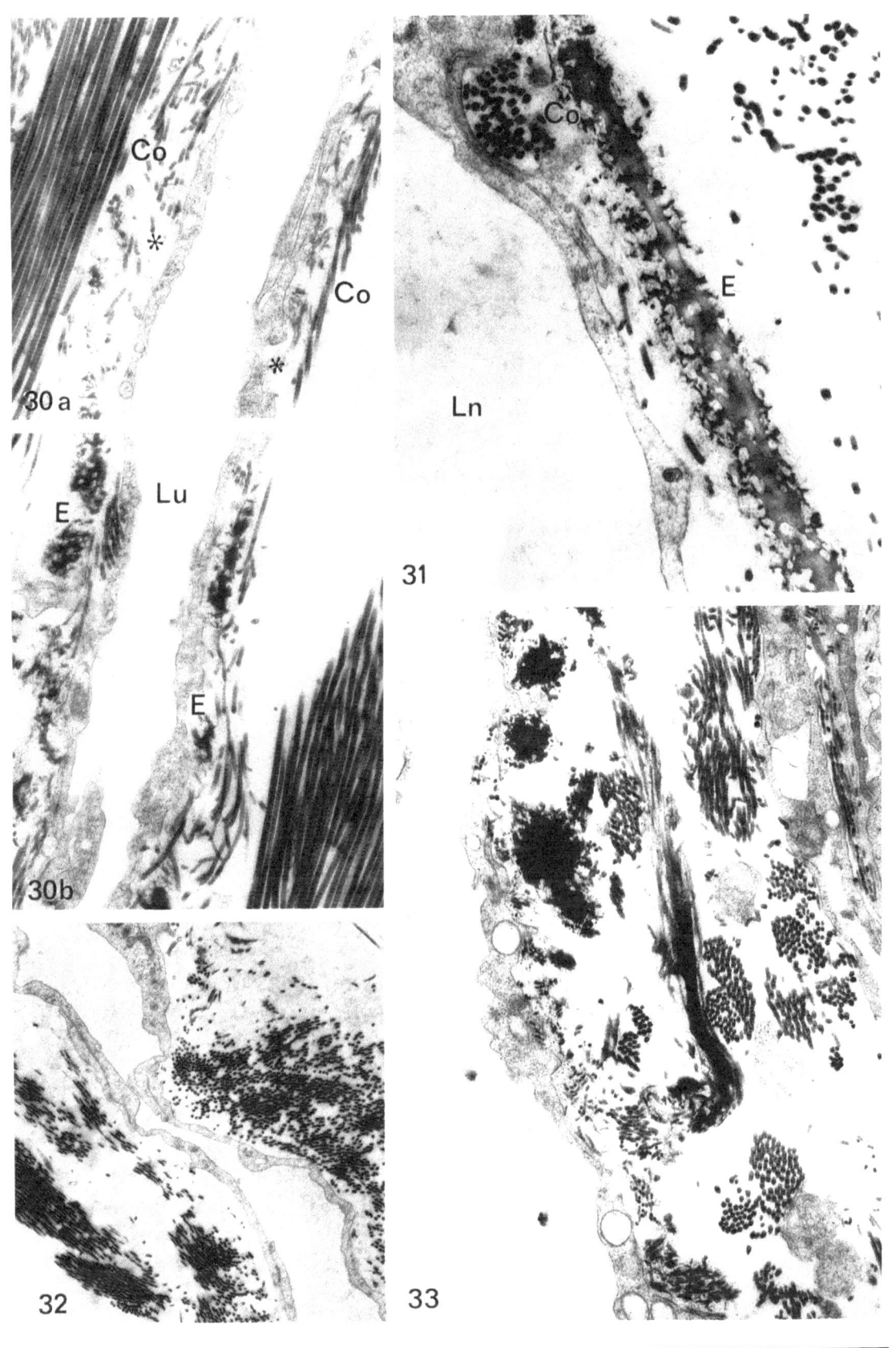

Fig. 34. Inflammation, eczematous rat paw skin. One-cell valve. The modified endothelial cell protruding into the lumen *(Lu)* of the lymphatic capillary has only a short junctional connection *(arrow)* with the adjacent endothelial cells. The cytoplasm of the bulging endothelial cell is full of microfilament 6–7 nm in diameter. The endothelial cell surface is prickled by small pseudopodia. *Bl* Basal lamina; × 9800

Fig. 35. Atrophic skin, human lower leg. The dermal lymphatic capillary is accompanied by basal lamina fragments *(Bl)* and is surrounded by collagen fibers of different caliber *(Co)*. The endothelial cell contains dense granules *(g)* and the perinuclear region is characterized by a loose network of fine microfilaments *(mf)* 4–6 nm in diameter. *Lu,* Lymphatic lumen; × 4500

Fig. 36. Inflammation, eczematous rat paw skin. Detail of the lymphatic capillary endothelial cell. The cytoplasm is very rich in organelles, and a massive bundle of filaments *(mf)* runs through the cytoplasm parallel with the luminal *(Lu)* surface. The filaments, 6–7 nm in diameter, display a longitudinal periodic striation. The cytoplasmic pseudopodia *(p)* protrude into the dermis. *ri,* Ribosomes; × 10000

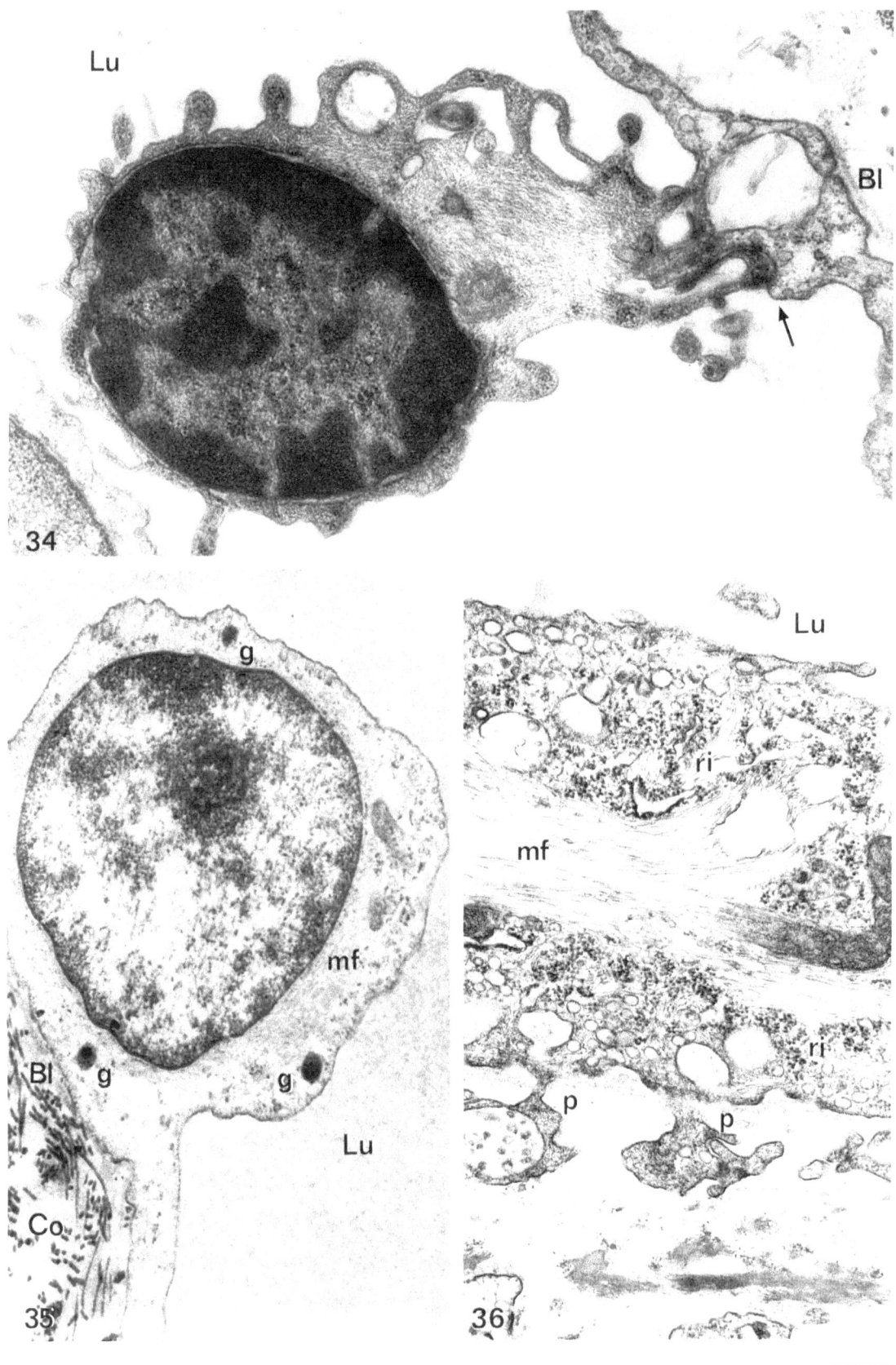

Fig. 37. Lymphedema, hyperkeratosis, human lower leg. Detail of the endothelial cell of a dermal lymphatic capillary. The cytoplasm contains pinocytotic vesciles *(v)*, mitochondria *(Mi)*, and a multivesicular body *(mvb)* surrounded by a unit membrane. × 30000

Fig. 38. Inflammation, eczematous rat paw skin. The pinocytotic vesicles are numerous at both the luminal *(Lu)* and abluminal surfaces. The Golgi apparatus *(Go)* is well developed; the longitudinal section of a perinuclear centriole *(Ce)* is seen. The basal lamina *(Bl)* is discontinuous. The number of dense cytoplasmic plates along the abluminal cell surface *(stars)* is increased. × 16000

Fig. 39. Inflammation, eczematous rat paw skin. A circumscribed region of the lymphatic endothelial cell bulging into the capillary lumen *(Lu)* contains a great number of dense mitochondria *(Mi)*. × 5000

Fig. 40. Inflammation, eczematous rat paw skin. Detail of lymphatic capillary endothelial cell. The cytoplasm contains Golgi cisternae *(Go)*, ribosomes *(ri)*, and numerous pinocytotic vesicles *(v)* around the lumen *(Lu)* and along the abluminal membrane surface. The perinuclear endoplasmic reticulum continues into a tetramembranous tubular complex *(arrow)* of the perinuclear endoplasmic reticulum *(Er)*. × 25000

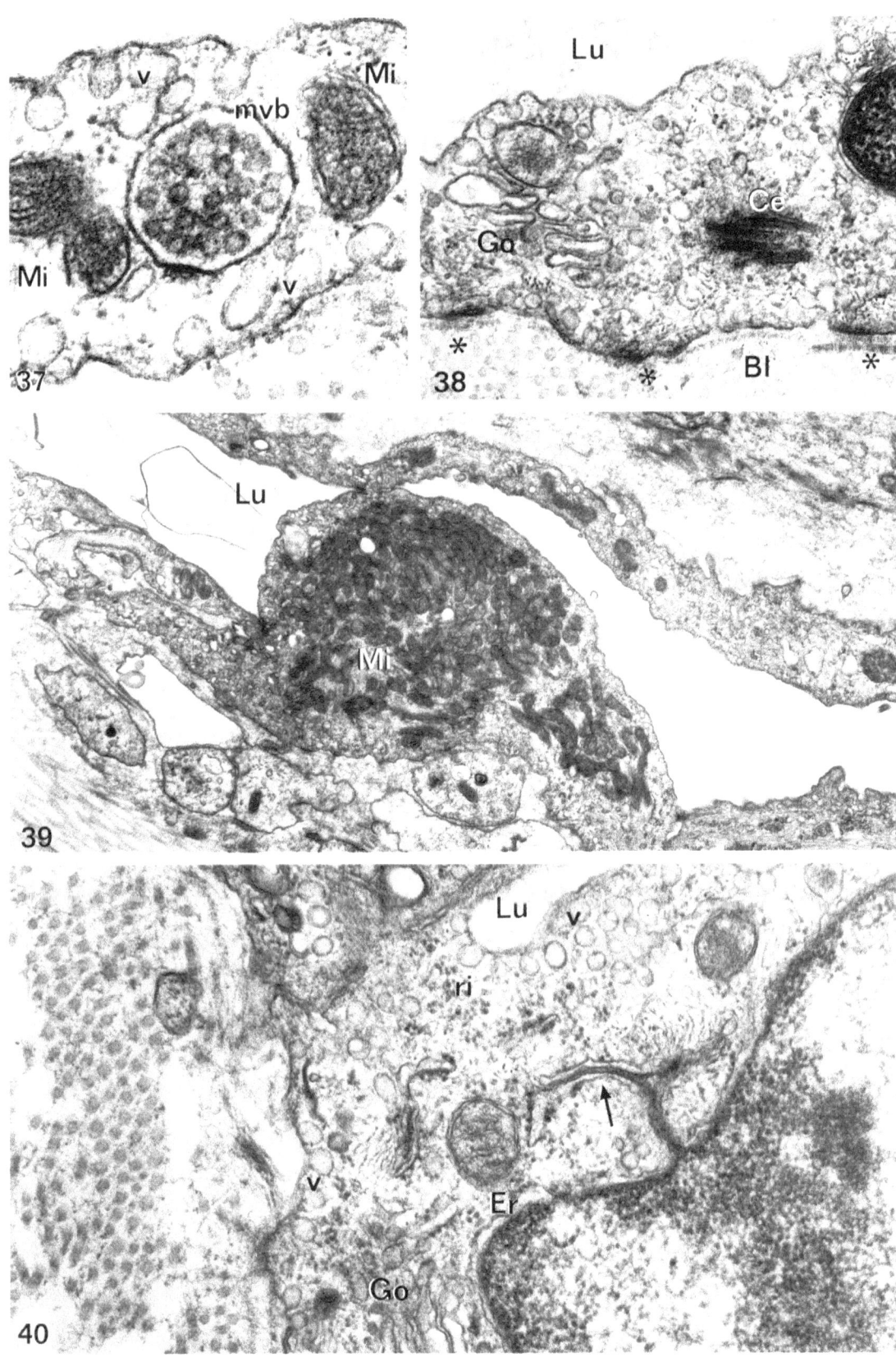

Fig. 41. Inflammation, eczematous rat paw skin. The most characteristic organelles in this lymphatic endothelial cell are the basal bodies of the cilia *(stars). Lu,* Lymphatic lumen; *Co,* collagen fibers; × 14000

Fig. 42. Lymphedema, canine hind limb. The overlapping and interdigitating endothelial cells of the lymphatic capillary display a perinuclear inclusion of tubuloreticular structures *(TRS)* and a lipid droplet *(Li)* surrounded by concentric membranes. *Lu,* Lymphatic lumen; × 12500

Fig. 43. Lymphedema, canine hind limb. Detail of a perilymphatic macrophage *(Ma)* with accordion-like wrinkling of cytoplasmic processes and large dense cytoplasmic inclusions of lipid substances *(stars)* in the cytoplasm. The perilymphatic connective tissue cell contains lipid droplets *(Li)* partly limited by a membrane. × 5500

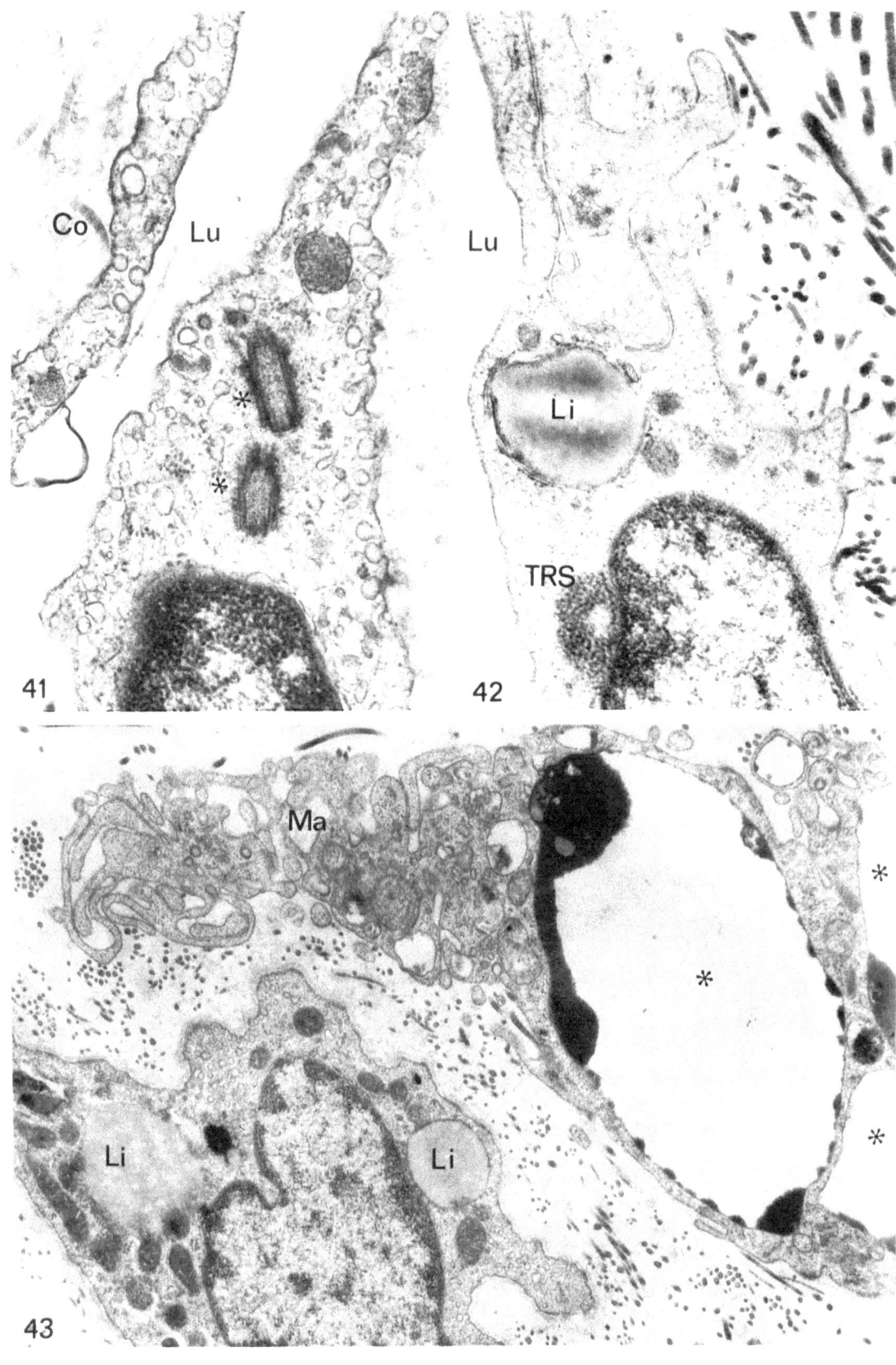

Fig. 44. Inflammation, eczematous rat paw skin. The cytoplasm of the endothelial cells surrounding the dilated lumina *(Lu)* of the lymphatic capillary looks like a sack full of pearls due to the large number of cytoplasmic vesicles. The collagen fibers *(Co)* are directly connected to the abluminal surface of the endothelial cells. × 5000

Fig. 45. Inflammation, eczematous rat paw skin. Detail of a dermal lymphatic capillary. One of the numerous pinocytotic vesicles possesses a diaphragm with a central knob *(arrow). Lu,* Lymphatic lumen; × 43000

Fig. 46. Inflammation, eczematous rat paw skin. The membranes of the pinocytotic vesicles can fuse with each other *(arrow),* and at the flat endothelial segment the vesicles can probably communicate with both the lumen *(Lu)* and the abluminal surface *(star).* The collagen fibers *(Co)* run directly to the endothelial cell membrane. × 12000

Fig. 47. Inflammation, eczematous rat paw skin. A tubular microfilament is seen in the endothelial coated vesicle *(star)* The anchoring tubular microfilaments are demonstrated *(arrow)* in the perilymphatic connective tissue. *Lu,* Lymphatic lumen; × 24000

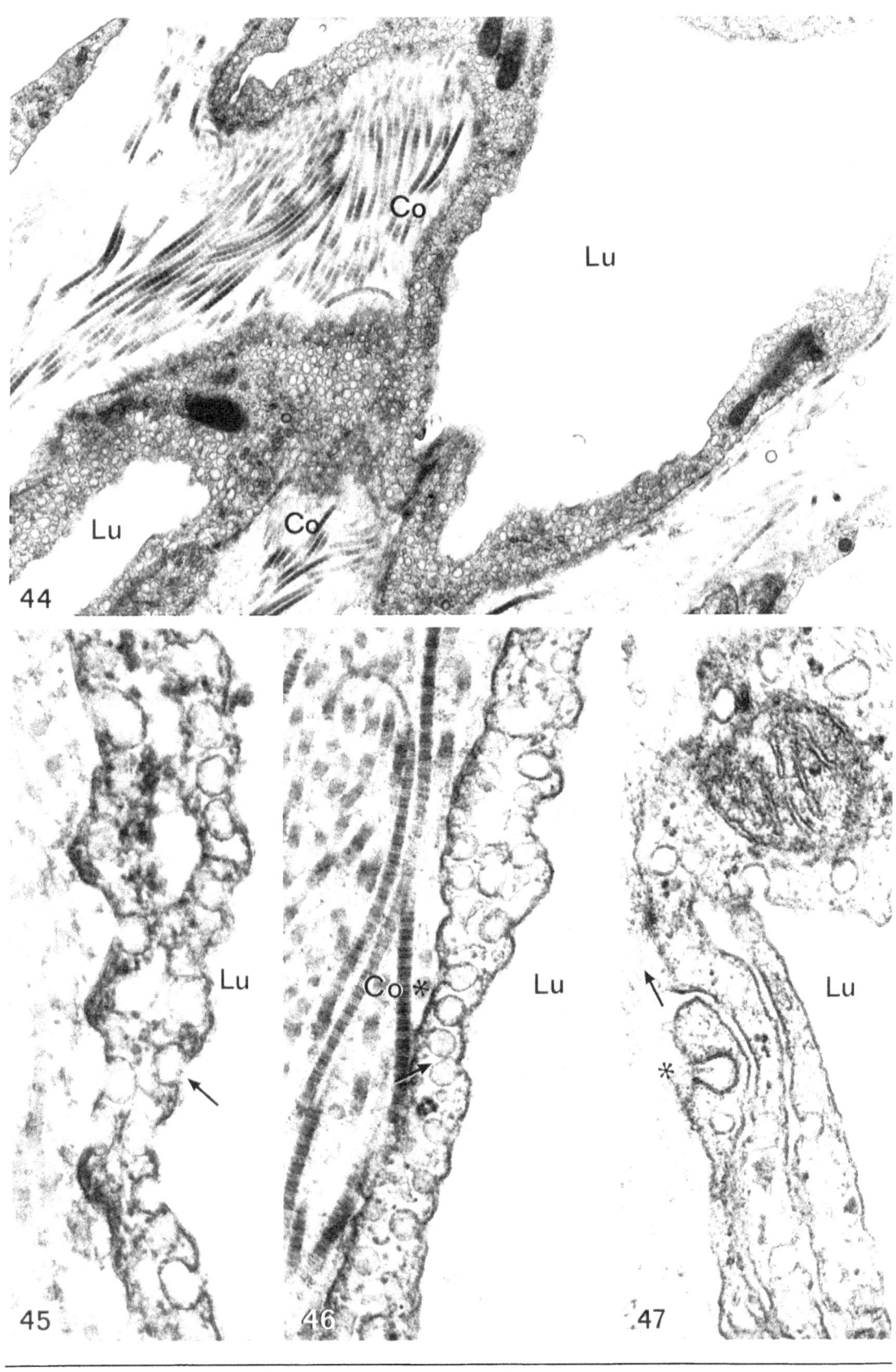

Fig. 48. Lymphedema, canine hind limb. Detail of a lymphatic capillary endothelial cell. The cytoplasm contains lysosomal inclusions *(star),* lipid droplets *(Li)* without a limiting membrane, and a paracrystalline arrangement of membranous tubules *(arrow)* located within the cisternae of endoplasmic reticulum. × 9800

Fig. 49. Lymphedema, canine hind limb. Two lymphatic capillaries *(Lu$_{1-2}$)* are seen in close vicinity. Numerous dense granules *(g)* are observed in the endothelial cytoplasm of the Lu$_1$ capillary. In the Lu$_2$ capillary endothelial cell the tubuloreticular *(TRS)* inclusion is composed of loosely aggregated tubules surrounded by a membrane. × 7200

Fig. 50. Human skin, systemic lupus erythematosus, forearm. The dilated lymphatic lumen *(Lu)* is full of fine granular and filamentous material. The narrow interstitial border around the capillary displays the same density where collagen fibers *(Co)* are intermingled with the dense granulofilamentous substance. In the endothelial cell a tubuloreticular inclusion *(arrow)* is observable. × 4800 *Inset:* Close-up of the tubuloreticular inclusion *(TRS)* composed of reticular aggregates of tubules within a membrane-bound vacuole. × 19000

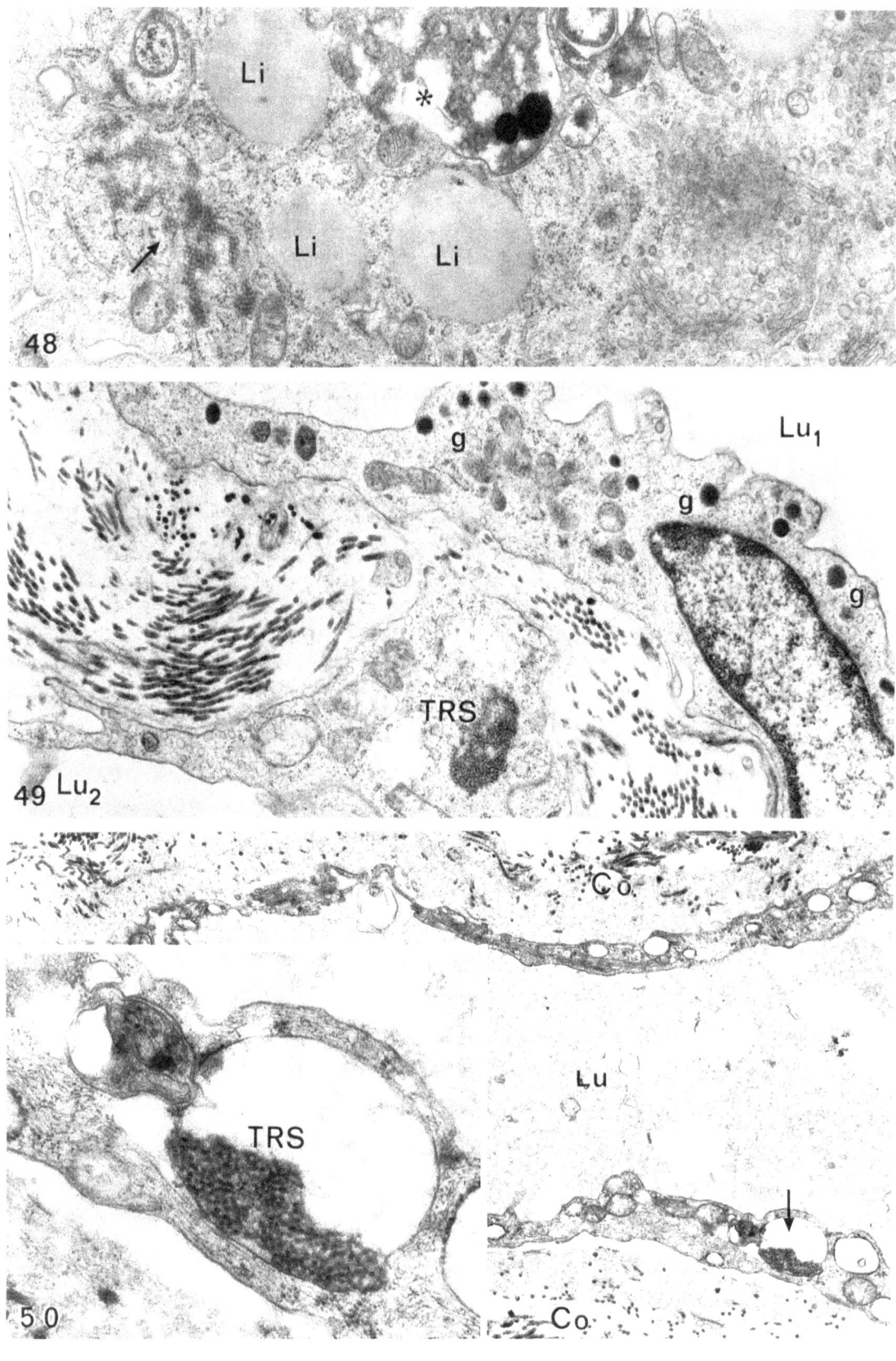

Fig. 51. Lymphedema, human lower leg. The nucleus of the lymphatic capillary endothelial cell has a prominent nucleolus *(nu)* and three granulofilamentous nuclear bodies *(nb)*. The nuclear blebs are bordered by a very slim bridge of the nucleoplasm *(arrows)*. The contents of the blebs display cytoplasmic features. *Lu,* Lymphatic lumen; × 7200

Fig. 52. Lymphedema, human lower leg. Nuclear pseudoinclusion of the lymphatic capillary endothelial cell contains membrane-bound phagosomes and myelin bodies *(star)*. The pseudoinclusion is surrounded by a nuclear membrane. On this section plane the cytoplasmic contents of the deep nuclear invagination appear to be situated within the nucleoplasm, *nb,* Nuclear body; *Lu,* lymphatic lumen; × 6400

Fig. 53. Lymphedema, human lower leg. Detail of lymphatic capillary endothelial cell. The intranuclear inclusion is surrounded by a clear halo *(star)* and a circular dense rim of the nucleoplasm. The nuclear inclusion looks like a target or an owl's eye. The concentric lamellae have different densities: three dense lamellae alternate with three lighter rings. The lamellae have fuzzy borders. × 15000

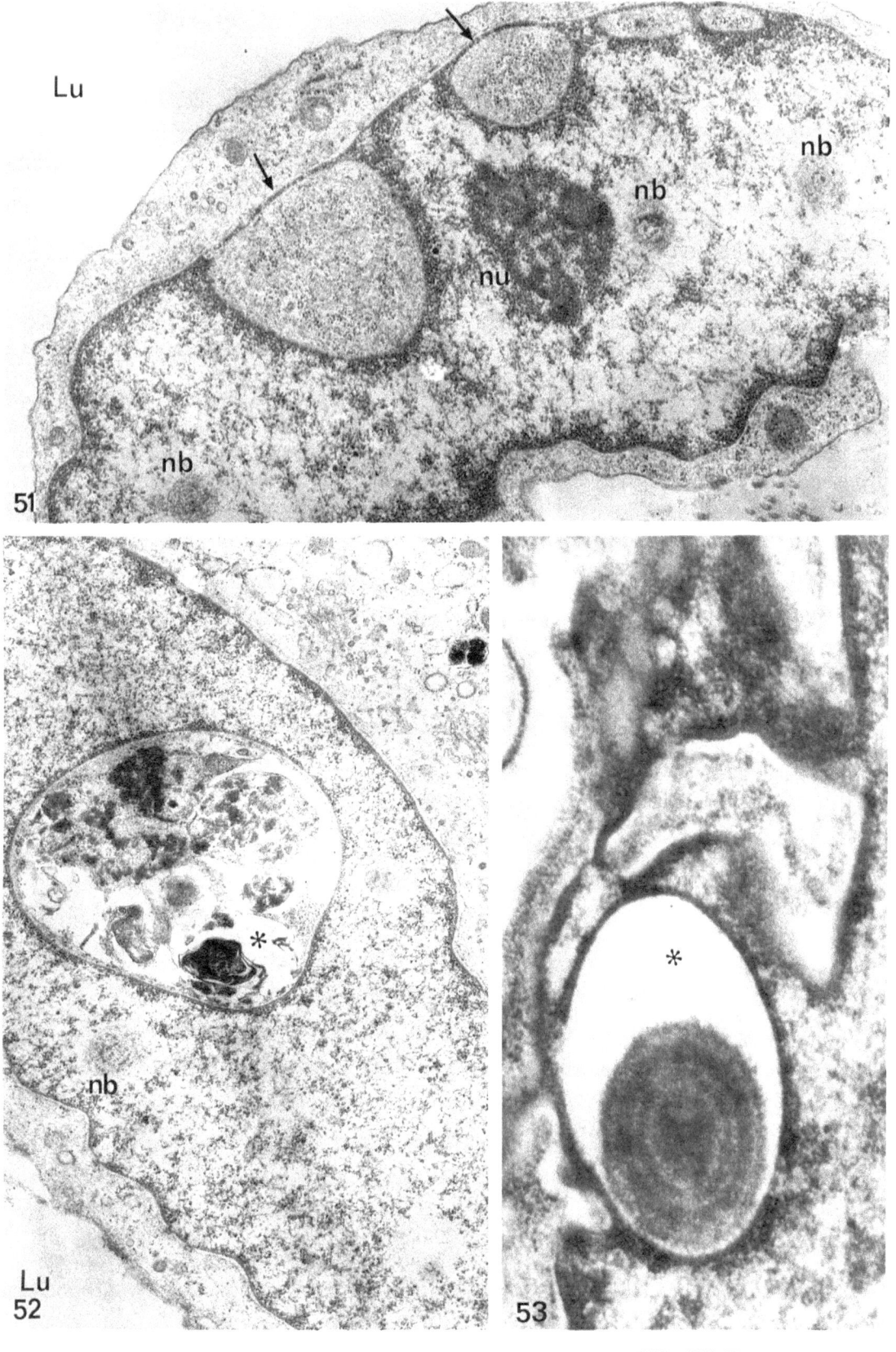

5 The Lymphatic Valve System

5.1 Structure of the Valves

The valves project into the lumen and are so arranged as to allow free passage of fluid and cells toward the larger lymphatic vessels. The arrangement of the valves prevents passage of fluid and cells in the reverse direction.

The most common form of the lymphatic valve is the bicuspid, but uni-, tri-, and quadricuspid forms were also encountered. The different types of valves can occur in combination and they vary greatly in appearance (DARÓCZY 1984c). Recognizing the real nature of the three-dimensional valve modulations on histological sections can be difficult (Figs. 54–56). Interpretation of the three-dimensional valve configurations remains a task that will hopefully be solved by a fortunate combination of diligent work and fantasy.

From isolated lymphatics (collecting lymphatic vessels) fixed in glutaraldehyde solution, GNEPP (1976) constructed a three-dimensional model on which he demonstrated the bicuspid nature of the valves. We have constructed a model based on our experience with serial sections. The three-dimensional model shows a bicuspid valve. (Fig. 57) Some section planes are indicated which would produce the conditions of the valves that we realized on the histological sections (Figs. 54–56, 58, 59).

The dermal lymphatic capillaries do possess valves. The valves are folds of the vessel wall. They have a connective tissue base and a connective tissue core that is covered on both sides by endothelial cells. This valvular endothelium is continuous with the endothelium of the wall (TAKADA 1971; VAJDA and TOMCSIK 1971).

5.1.1 Connective Tissue

The connective tissue "backbone" of the valve, bulging into the lumen or bridging it, consists of collagen, elastic fibers, and microfilaments (Figs. 60–62). The connective tissue core of the valve is continuous with the perivascular connective tissue (Figs. 61, 64). In some portions of the valve thick bundles of the elastic microtubules can be detected running parallel with the long axis of the cusp. The microtubules measure 10–12 nm in diameter and show an irregular longitudinal periodicity of 10–12 nm (Fig. 63); they can be arranged in bundles. The microfilaments are attached to the cytoplasmic dense plates of the abluminal endothelial membrane.

Fibroblasts are rarely detected in the connective tissue stem of the valvular cusp (Fig. 64).

5.1.2 Basal Lamina

The basal lamina along the valvular endothelial cells is not continuous, but it can be prominent in some regions (Figs. 62–64).

5.1.3 Endothelial Cells

Valvular endothelial cells bulging into the lumen are usually flat with a rod-shaped nucleus (Fig. 62). They directly join the wall endothelium (Figs. 61, 64).

There were no differences in organelle contents between wall and valvular endothelial cells. The valvular endothelial cells were rich in cytoplasmic vesicles, but vesicles facing the lumen or the connective tissue have never been provided with a diaphragm. The cytoplasm of the valvular endothelial cells contains numerous filaments (TAKADA 1971). The filaments are randomly arranged and may serve a contractile function. They are 6–9 nm in diameter and their contractile properties are needed for movement of the valvular cusps to expand and contract for the passage of fluid and prevent regurgitation.

Along the free edge of the valvular cusp the endothelial cells budding into the lumen are distinguishable from other endothelial cells (LEAK 1972; TAKADA 1971). These tip cells have short connections with the valvular connective tissue that are characterized by well-developed basal lamina segments and numerous dense cytoplasmic attachment plates (Figs. 65–70).

The nuclei of the tip cells can be oval but they are mainly elongated and rod-shaped with an indented contour. Their long axes are parallel with the long axis of the lymphatic lumen and they protrude into the lumen like arrowheads directed into the proximal segment. Nucleoli and nuclear bodies are very rare.

The narrow cytoplasmic rim around the nucleus is rich in ribosomes; mitochondria, smooth-surfaced endoplasmic tubules, and vesicles along the luminal surface can be revealed (Figs. 64, 70).

The tip cells may be connected by cytoplasmic junctions sealing the lymphatic segments. The elongated pseudopodia-like cytoplasmic processes of the tip cells may also create junctions with each other or with the neighbouring tip cells (Figs. 68–70). The number of tip cells varies, the nuclei bulging into the lumen are sometimes numerous (Fig. 67).

5.2 Main Forms of the Lymphatic Valves

Four types of valves have been observed (DARÓCZY 1984a, b): joining valves, segment valves, unicellular valves, and bunch valves.

5.2.1 Joining Valves

The joining valve is detectable at the point where lymphatics join one another. These valves contain a core of connective tissue that is connected with the perivascular connective tissue and covered by endothelial cells which join directly with the wall endothelium. The organelle content of the valvular endothelial cells is the same as that of the wall endothelial cells. The attachment plates between the connective tissue and the endothelial cells of the valve are more numerous than in the wall and the basal lamina is discontinuous. There are no open intercellular junctions along the valvular endothelium. At the edges of the valve cusps, tip cells display morphological properties distinguishable from other endothelial cells; i.e., they bud into the lumen, have indented rod-shaped nuclei, make short connections with the connective tissue backbone of the cusp, and have pseudopodia-like elongated projections. The number of tip cells varies from one to five (Figs. 65 and 66). The tip cells can be connected with each other by membrane junctions sealing the lumen.

5.2.2 Segment Valves

Segment valves consist of folds of connective tissue which extend into the lumen and divide the vessel into discrete segments. The segment valves emanate from facing walls. The luminal surface of the valve is covered by endothelial cells connected directly with the wall endothelium.

There are no differences in organelle content between wall and valvular endothelial cells.

Well-developed segments of basal lamina and short attachment plates are seen along the junctional zone between the connective tissue and endothelial cells of the cusp. The tip cells have elongated processes, and they are able to seal the luminal segments due to junctions between the adjoining cells. The number of tip cells varies from one to four (Figs. 67–70).

The distance between the segment valves varies, probably depending on the segment studied and on the stage of activity. It is not common to be able to demonstrate three to four pairs of valves on the same section, but this situation is very helpful in analyzing the construction of the valves and in interpreting their three-dimensional features (Figs. 71–73). The three pairs of valves seen in the dilated lumen of the lymphatic capillary were serially cut and the different configurations of the sections were analyzed. The valvular cusps seem either to be open or to seal the segment, or they look like elongated connective-tissue folds crossing through the lumen (Fig. 71 a).

The serial sections allow construction of a three-dimensional model presenting two pairs of valves and a single cusp (Fig. 72). The construction of a three-dimensional model was the result of an analytical study. We cut the model through an indicated section plane to demonstrate that the model represents the original condition of the valve structures seen on histological sections (Fig. 73). The reverse process, cutting the three-dimensional model in order to produce the situation of the histological sections, confirms the reality of the model.

Estimation of the real configurations of the valves on the histological sections is very difficult because of the numerous possible appearances of valvular cusps and valvular endothelial cells. Only consecutive histological sections can demonstrate the real situation of the valvular structures (DARÓCZY 1984 a; Figs. 74–77). If the section plane runs through the basal portion of the cusp from the pair of valves, this single section can imitate a temporary valve produced by connective tissue protrusion (Fig. 78). The three-dimensional model demonstrates and helps to understand how the section plane of one cusp can lead to misinterpretation of the valvular structure (Figs. 79 and 80).

5.2.3 Unicellular Valves

This type of valves is formed by a single endothelial cell separated in part from neighbouring endothelial cells bulging into the lumen (DARÓCZY 1984 a). It extends deeply into the lumen while maintaining connections with adjacent

wall endothelial cells. The contact with the perivascular connective tissue is short and escorted by dense cytoplasmic attachment plates and prominent segments of basal lamina (Fig. 81). The junctional structures are better developed here than in other parts of the wall. This unique modified endothelial cell projects like a short bud into the lumen (DARÓCZY 1982).

The shape of these intraluminal-appearing endothelial cells varies; they can be oval, round, or rod-shaped. The nuclei of the unicellular valves also vary, being indented, oval, or spindle-shaped. Sometimes the modified endothelial cells span the lumen to approach the endothelium of the opposite side (Fig. 81).

The surface of the budding cell can be smooth or it can display prickles or longer pseudopodia projecting into the lumen. The cytoplasm contains short tubules of rough-surfaced endoplasmic reticulum, free ribosomes, mitochondria, vesicles along the luminal surface, and abundant filaments 6–9 nm in diameter. They are often bundled at the cell base of the valve, in the narrow neck of the modified cell (Figs. 81 and 82) or around the nucleus of the protruding endothelial cell (Fig. 83).

Unicellular valves have been observed by other investigators and described as single flaps of the lymphatic endothelium protruding into the lumen (VAJDA and TOMCSIK 1971) or as lamellar endothelial projections budding from the lymphatic wall (PAPP et al. 1962).

5.2.4 Bunch Valves

The stem of the bunch consists of a connective-tissue fold connected directly with the perivascular interstitium and covered by a single layer of endothelial cells that are connected with the wall endothelium. Along its free edge, endothelial cells budding into the lumen like flowers in a bunch differ from other endothelial cells (DARÓCZY 1983 a–c). These are modified endothelial cells, the so-called tip cells (Fig. 84). They have extremely short connections with the connective-tissue components of the valvular backbone. This junctional area is characterized by well-developed cytoplasmic attachment plates and prominent segments of basal lamina (Fig. 85).

Intercellular tight junctions between adjoining tip cells are also encountered. Open intercellular junctions (gaps) were not visible at the bunch-valve region.

The shape of tip cells varies, being oval, spindle-shaped, or pedunculated. Nuclei of the modified endothelial cells also varies, being oval or drop-shaped, with smooth or indented surfaces (Figs. 84 and 85).

The tip cells have elongated pseudopodia-like projections and the cells float in the lumen of the lymphatic capillary. Their cytoplasm is rich in 6- to 9-nm filaments. Both the cross sections (at the base of the tip cell) and longitudinal sections (around the nucleus) of the cytoplasmic filaments can be observed due to the network-like arrangement of the filaments (Figs. 85 and 86). In our material the highest number of budding tip cells was seven; however, nuclei were detected only on serial sections (DARÓCZY 1984 b).

The bunch-valve structures were described by LEAK (1972 a) without comment. The folds of endothelial cells were separated by a delicate meshwork of connective-tissue elements consisting of collagen fibers and occasional fibroblasts. Along the free edge of the connective-tissue stem the endothelial cells were budding into the lumen.

5.3 Inlet Valves

Intercellular gaps in the lymphatic endothelial wall are usually observable. The endothelial cells can move across each other and they can also move away from each other, creating the open junctions along the capillary wall. The gaps can appear due to:

1. A pulling mechanism of the perivascular connective tissue (microfilaments of the connective tissue, elastic and collagen fibers)
2. Passive movement of the perivascular connective tissue (due to massage, pulsation of the arteries, respiratory forces, muscle contractions, etc.)
3. Active contractions of the endothelial cells

The interendothelial open junctions act as inlet valves (CASLEY-SMITH 1964 a). The inlet valves are of great importance for the quick transport of fluid and materials through the lymphatic wall. The junctions between the overlapping flaps of endothelial cells are open over only part of their length. An intraendothelial channel is constructed between two cytoplasmic processes of neighbouring endothelial cells if the abluminal cytoplasmic projection envelops a subendothelial space before joining the adjacent endothelial cell. The three-dimensional model shows a partly closed lymphatic capillary segment with an open junction between the flaps of the adjacent endothelial cells (Fig. 87).

AZZALI (1982) demonstrated the lock-gate mechanism of the temporary intraendothelial channels and constructed a three-dimensional model to confirm the opening and closing movements of the endothelial processes due to the endothelial rearrangements. With serial sections one can interpret the anatomical situations and reconstruct the real morphological conditions (Fig. 88).

The funnel-like valves (LAUWERYNS 1971) and the endothelial cell processes protruding into the capillary lumen can produce on the section plane a "lumen-in-lumen" appearance. The serial sections helped to reconstruct the special anatomical situation. The smaller capillary joining a larger lymphatic vessel, on the histological section, seems to float in the lumen of the larger lymphatic. The cutting plane through the model demonstrated the joining capillary as a "lumen in lumen" of the larger vessel (Figs. 89–91).

The interendothelial channels enveloped by endothelial cell processes may represent lock-gate chambers which are temporarily closed but may be opened into the lymphatic lumen or into the interstitium. In this way the perivascular space may be directly connected with a part of the lumen that is surrounded by elongated processes of the endothelial cells (Fig. 92).

The inlet valve is formed by endothelial cell processes which can overlap each other, and only the serial sections revealed the gap between the adjacent cells (Figs. 93 and 94).

The overlapping areas of the neighbouring

wall endothelial cells were analyzed by serial sectioning (COLLAN and KALIMA 1974). The series showed that the endothelial cells changed their positions in relation both to one another and to the lumen of the lymphatic capillary. The closed areas might change into open ones and vice versa.

The inlet valves and the intraendothelial channels of the lymphatic capillaries play an important role for the drainage function of the capillaries.

The interendothelial space closed by tight junctions was labeled by lanthanum nitrate. The perivascular space did not contain any contrast material (Fig. 95). Tight junctions do exist between the adjacent endothelial cells which seal the intercellular spaces, but it is suggested that the tight junctions may be rearranged, and in another stage loose connections can be visualized between the overlapping cell processes.

Intravenously injected ferritin particles appeared in the interstitium. They were seen as individual particles among the interstitial fibers, or they were shown as small groups in the interstitium. Some ferritin particles were demonstrated in the endothelial vesicles and in the lymphatic lumen (Fig. 96). The open junction in the lymphatic endothelial wall produced direct contact between the capillary lumen and the interstitium. The lanthanum poured into the interstitium and appeared in large patches around the open junctions (Fig. 97). Through the gap between the endothelial cell processes different cells can move through the capillary wall (Figs. 98 and 99).

Fig. 54. Normal human dermis, lower leg. Section plane no. I from serial sections demonstrates the discontinuity *(arrows)* of the elastic fibers surrounding the lymphatic capillary. The bicuspid valves are cut vertically to the long axis of the tip cells' bridge over the lumen. Orcein, × 120

Fig. 55. Section plane no. II (from the same series as in Fig. 54) shows that the elastic fibers do not form a lamina elastica; the elastic coat is discontinuous *(arrows)* and the fibers run parallel with the lymphatic wall or vertically *(E)* to it. The sails of the valves bridge over the lumen. Orcein, × 120

Fig. 56. Section plane no. III (from the same series as in Figs. 54 and 55) shows the tips of the bicuspid segment valve floating free in the capillary lumen. Orcein, × 120

Fig. 57. The three-dimensional model shows a bicuspid valve. The section planes indicated by lines I, II, and III are those illustrated in Figs. 54, 55, and 56 and on the models in Figs. 58 and 59

Fig. 58. The two pieces of the model are produced by cutting along the section lines I (upper piece) and II (lower piece) of the model in Fig. 57. These cutting surfaces correspond to histological conditions of Figs. 54 and 55.

Fig. 59. Section line III on the model in Fig. 57), running parallel with the direction *(arrow)* of the lymph flow, shows the "backbone" of the valve that is connected with the lymphatic wall *(arrowheads)* and the tip cells *(stars)* floating free in the lumen as seen in histological section of Fig. 56.

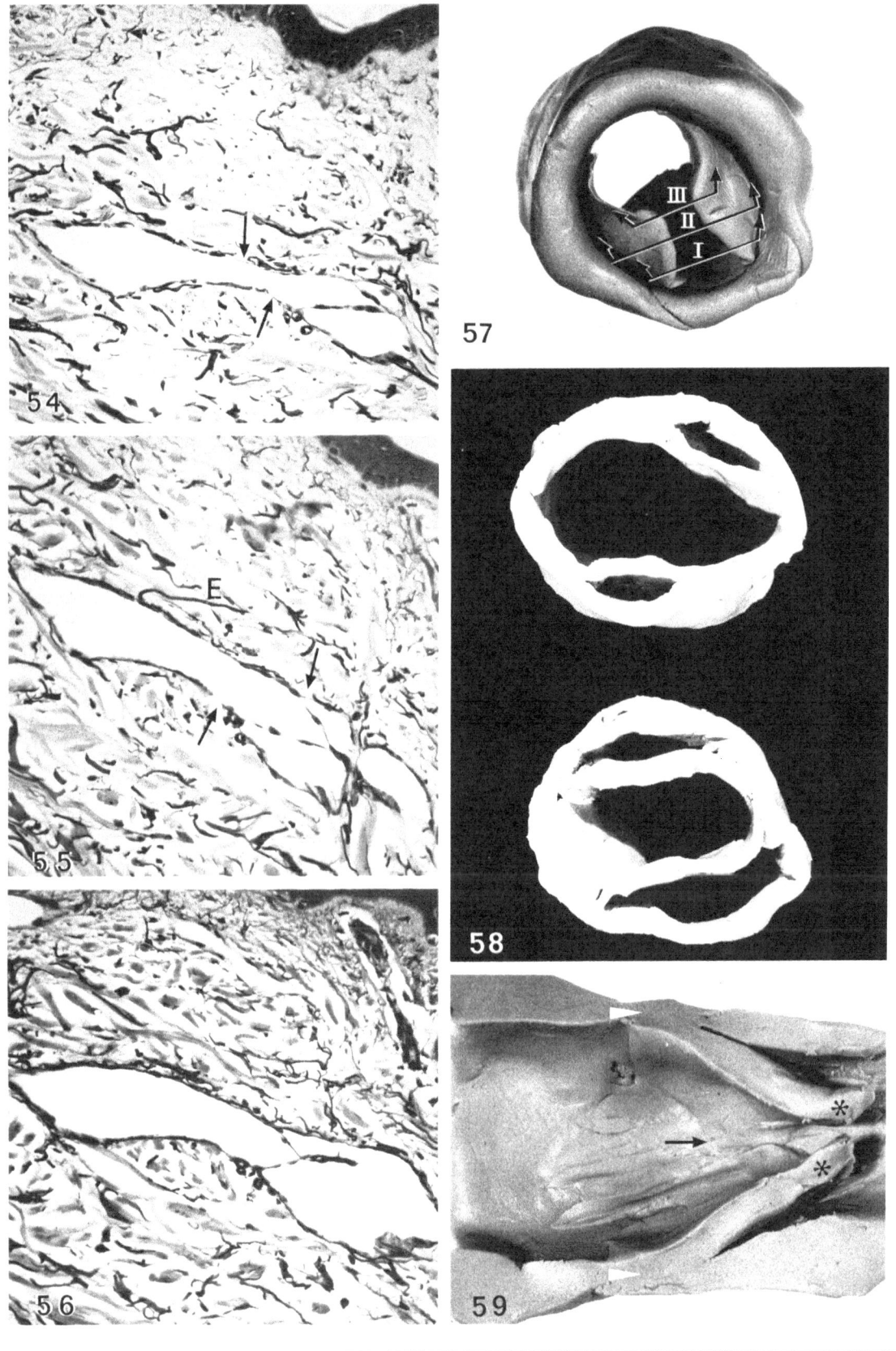

Fig. 60. Inflammation, eczematous rat paw skin. The dilated dermal lymphatic capillary is dissected into two parts by a valve cusp consisting of a connective tissue core covered by endothelial cells; in the lumen *(Lu)* an erythrocyte is present. Semithin section; toluidine blue, × 1000

Fig. 61. Human normal skin, lower leg. The valve (cut vertically to the lymph flow) bridges over the lymphatic capillary lumen *(Lu)*. The core of the cusp consists of connective tissue that is connected with the perivascular space. The endothelial cells covering the valvular connective tissue are in direct contact with the wall endothelium *(End)*. × 2500

Fig. 62. Inflammation, eczematous rat paw skin. The detail of a valvular cusp, dissecting into two parts the lymphatic capillary lumen *(Lu)* that contains erythrocytes, shows the connective tissue core, consisting of microfilaments and collagen fibers, and the endothelial cells *(End$_{1-2}$)* covering the surface of the cusp. × 5000

Fig. 63. Inflammation, eczematous rat paw skin. Close-up of the valvular connective tissue core covered by endothelium *(End$_{1-2}$)* on both sides. The microfilaments measuring 10–12 nm in diameter have a longitudinal periodicity. *Co,* Collagen fiber; × 24000

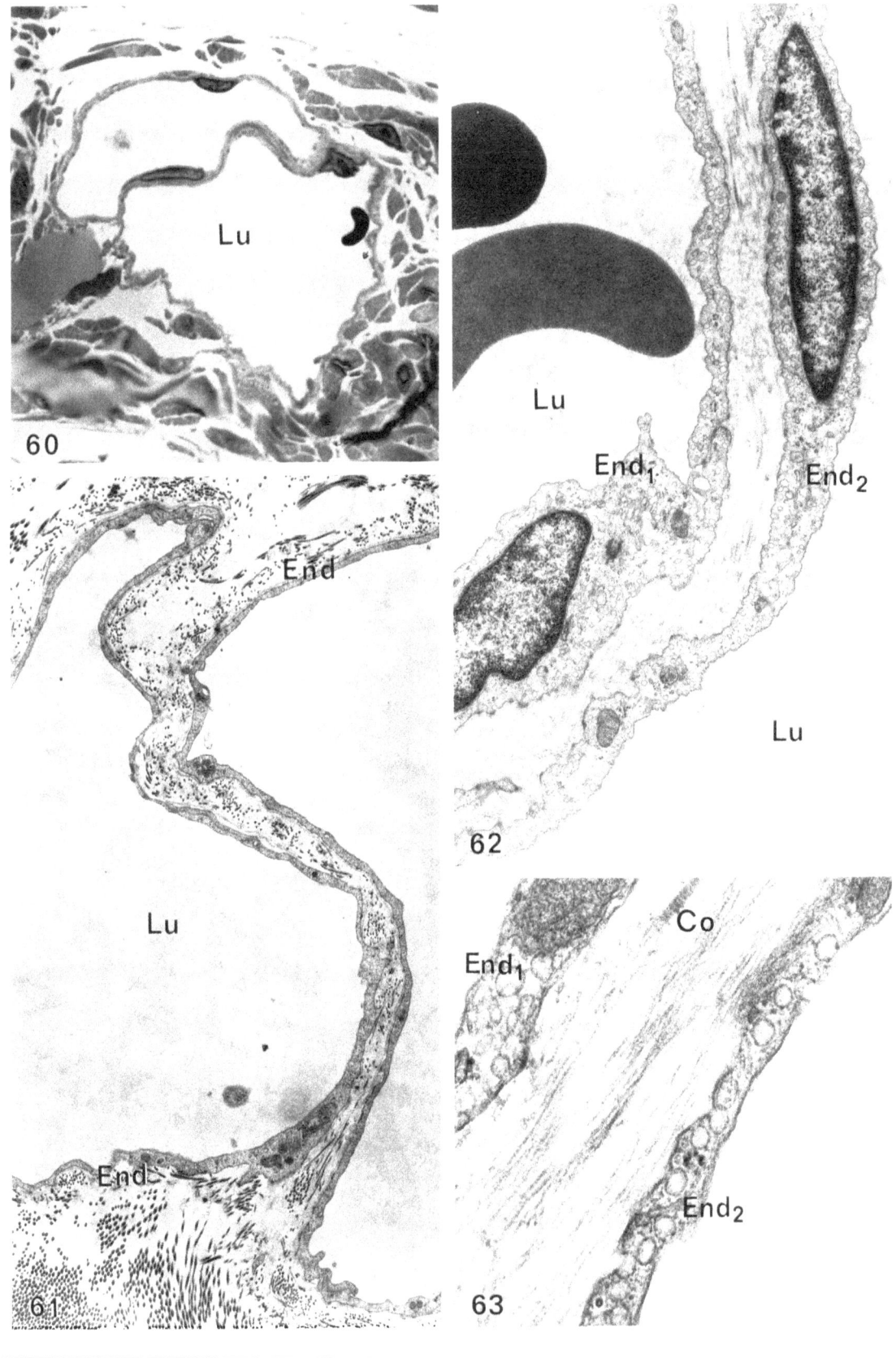

Fig. 64. Normal skin, canine hind limb. Montage of a lymphatic valvular cusp consisting of a connective tissue backbone containing microfilaments, collagen fibers *(Co)*, a fibroblast *(F)*, and a surface of endothelial cells joining directly with the wall endothelium *(stars)*. The tip cell of the valvular cusp turning back to the core of the valve *(arrow)* seems to be flexible. The attenuated endothelial wall of the lymphatic capillary is directly connected with the connective tissue. A continuous basal lamina is missing. × 4000

Fig. 64 □ 55

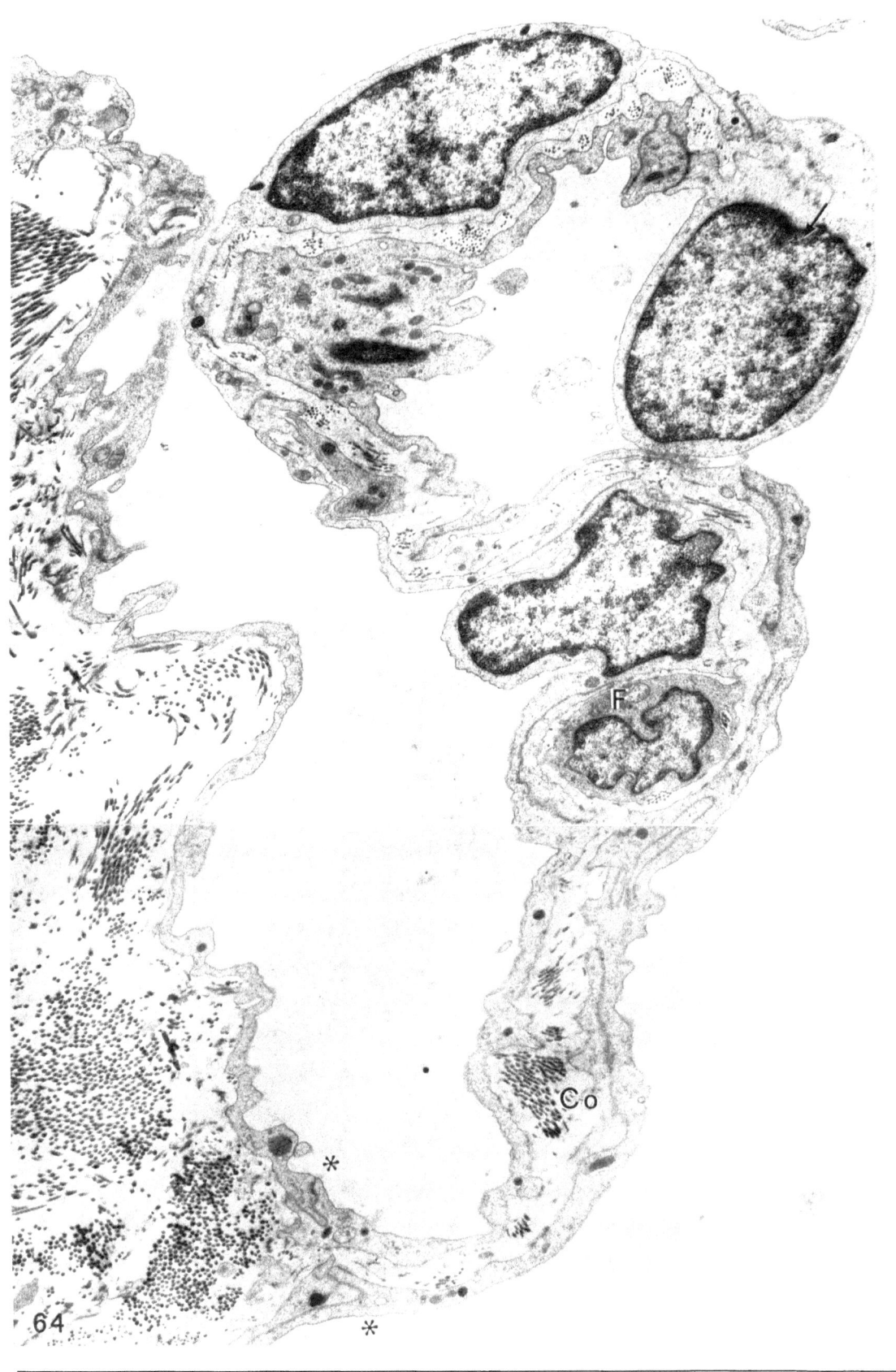

64

Fig. 65. Inflammation, eczematous rat paw skin. Two pairs *(A* and *B)* of joining valves are seen at the point where lymphatics join one another *(Lu₁* and *Lu₂)*. The joining valves contain a connective tissue core connected with the perivascular connective tissue *(arrows)* and a surface of endothelial cells joining directly with the wall enothelium *(End)*. The valvular tip cells bud into the lumen *(stars)*. × 1950

Fig. 66. Inflammation, eczematous rat paw skin. Semithin section of two pairs *(A* and *B)* of joining valves shown electron-microscopically in Fig. 65. The core of the valvular cusp consists of connective tissue folds *(arrows)* covered by endothelial cells which bud into the lumen along the free edge of the cusp *(stars)*. Toluidine blue, × 1000

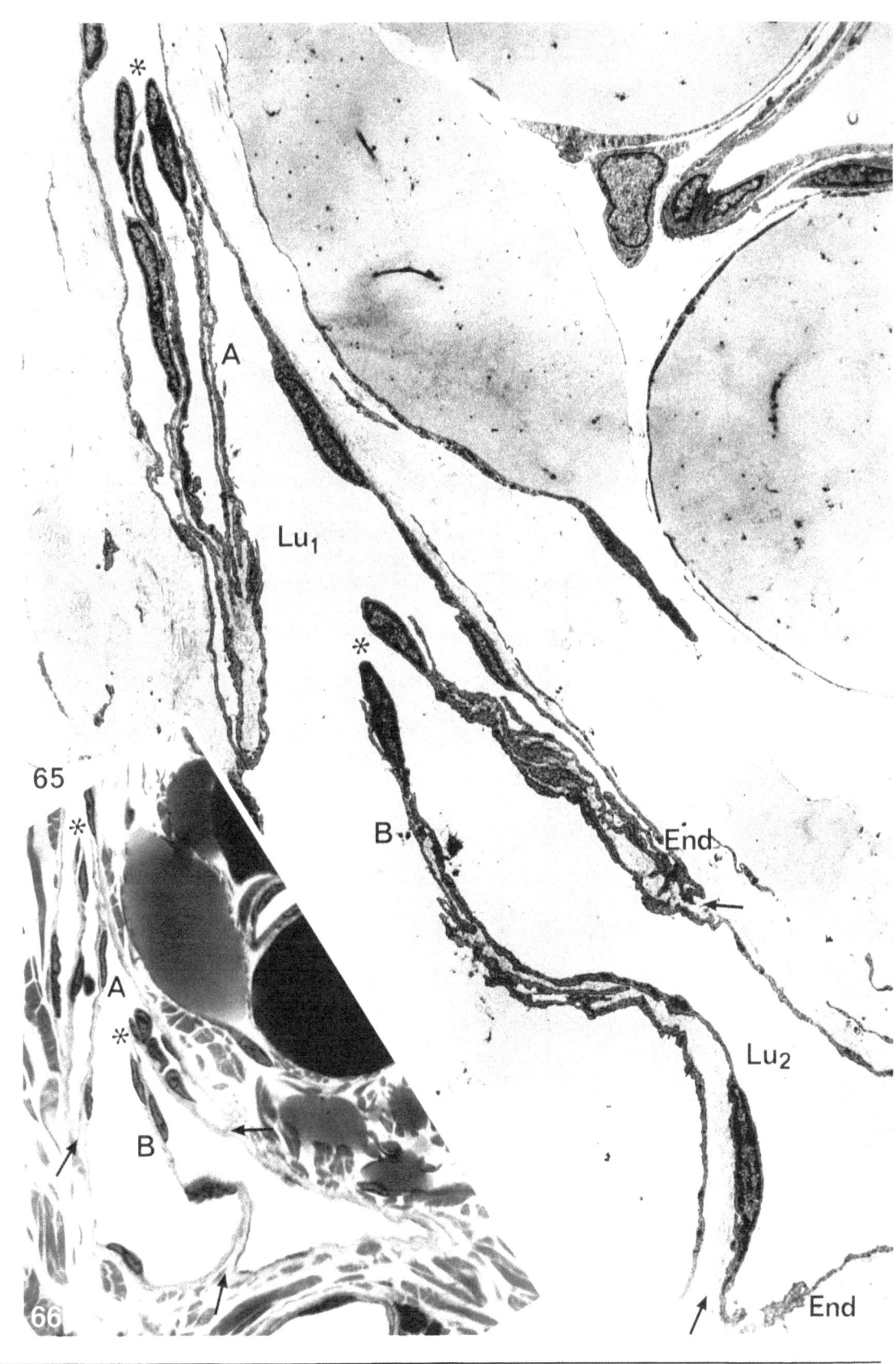

Fig. 67. Inflammation, eczematous rat paw skin. A segment valve divides the lumen into discrete segments. The tip cells *(star)* are very prominent. Semithin section; toluidine blue, × 500

Fig. 68. Inflammation, eczematous rat paw skin. The lumen is divided *(Lu$_{1-2}$)* by a segment valve consisting of folds of connective tissue which extend into the lumen *(star)*. The luminal surfaces of the cusps are covered by endothelial cells joining directly with the wall endothelium *(arrows)*. The endothelial cells budding into the lumen along the free edge of the cusps are the tip cells *(Tc)*. × 1950

Fig. 69. Close-up of the tip cells in Fig. 68. The tip cells seal the lymphatic lumen due to the junctions between them *(arrow)*. × 5000

Fig. 70. Inflammation, eczematous rat paw skin. The tip cells of the valve are characterized by elongated indented nuclei and pseudopodia-like cytoplasmic projections. The intercellular junctions between the adjoining tip cells *(arrows)* are able to seal the lymphatic segments. × 5000

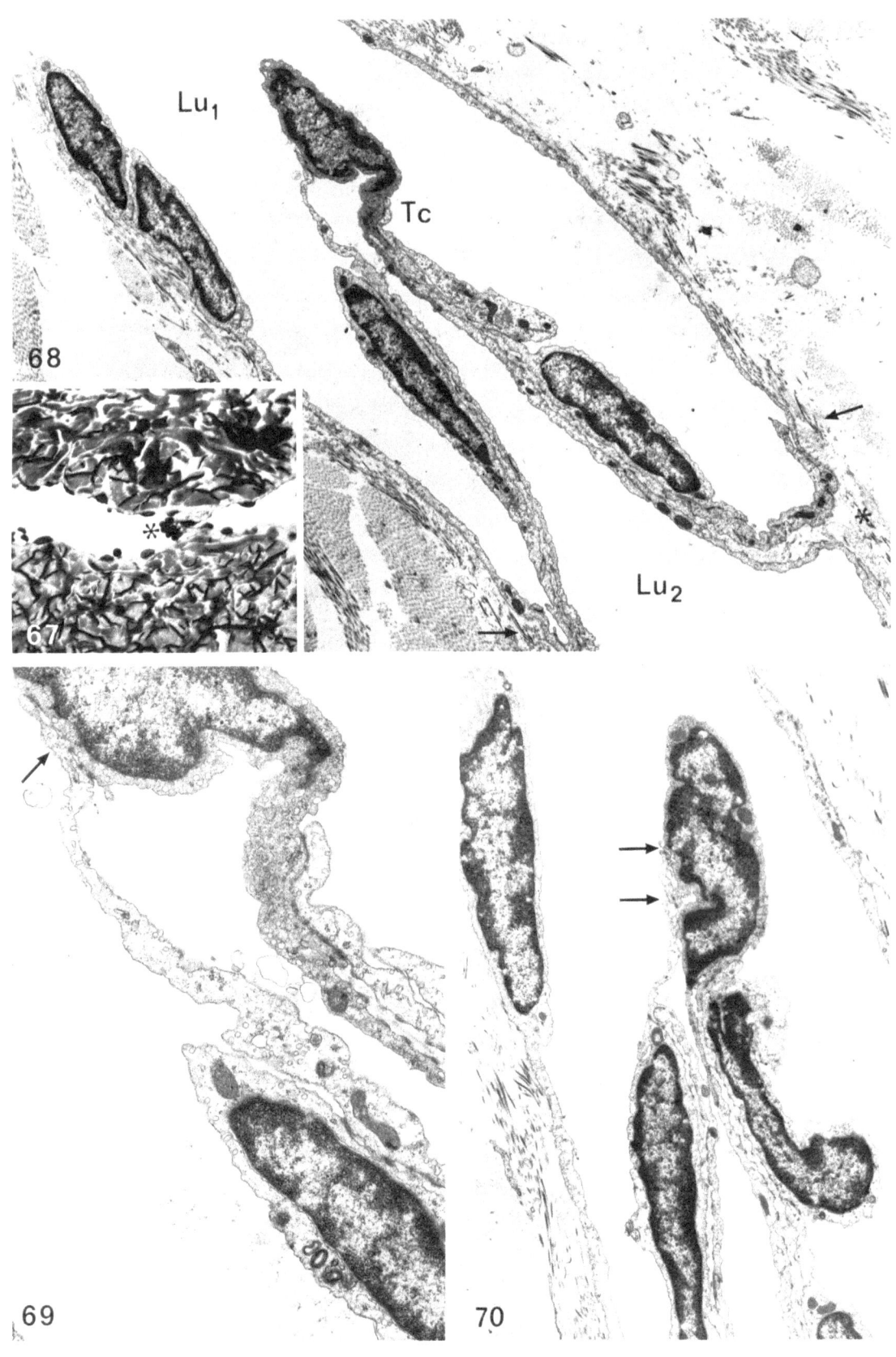

68

Lu₁

Tc

67

Lu₂

69

70

Fig. 71 a, b. Inflammation, eczematous rat paw skin.

a Three pairs of valves are seen in the dilated star-shaped lumen of the lymphatic capillary. One of them *(A)* seems to seal the lymphatic segment, the next one *(B)* is an open bicuspid valve, and the third *(C)* looks like elongated connective tissue processes. Semithin section; toluidine blue, × 500

b Close-up of the B and C valves. The processes of the B valvular tip cells are bulging into the lumen *(Lu)*. The C valve has elongated and convoluted cusps. In some folds *(stars)* of the lumen the lymph content is stained darker than in other places. × 800

Fig. 72. The model of the lymphatic capillary presented in Fig. 71. The three-dimensional model shows two pairs of valves *(A* and *B)* and one single cusp *(C)*. The plane of the section demonstrated in Figs. 71 and 73 is indicated by an *arrow*.

Fig. 73. A model of the lymph vessel section of Fig. 71, showing the two bicuspid valves *(A* and *B)* and the loop of the *C* cusp

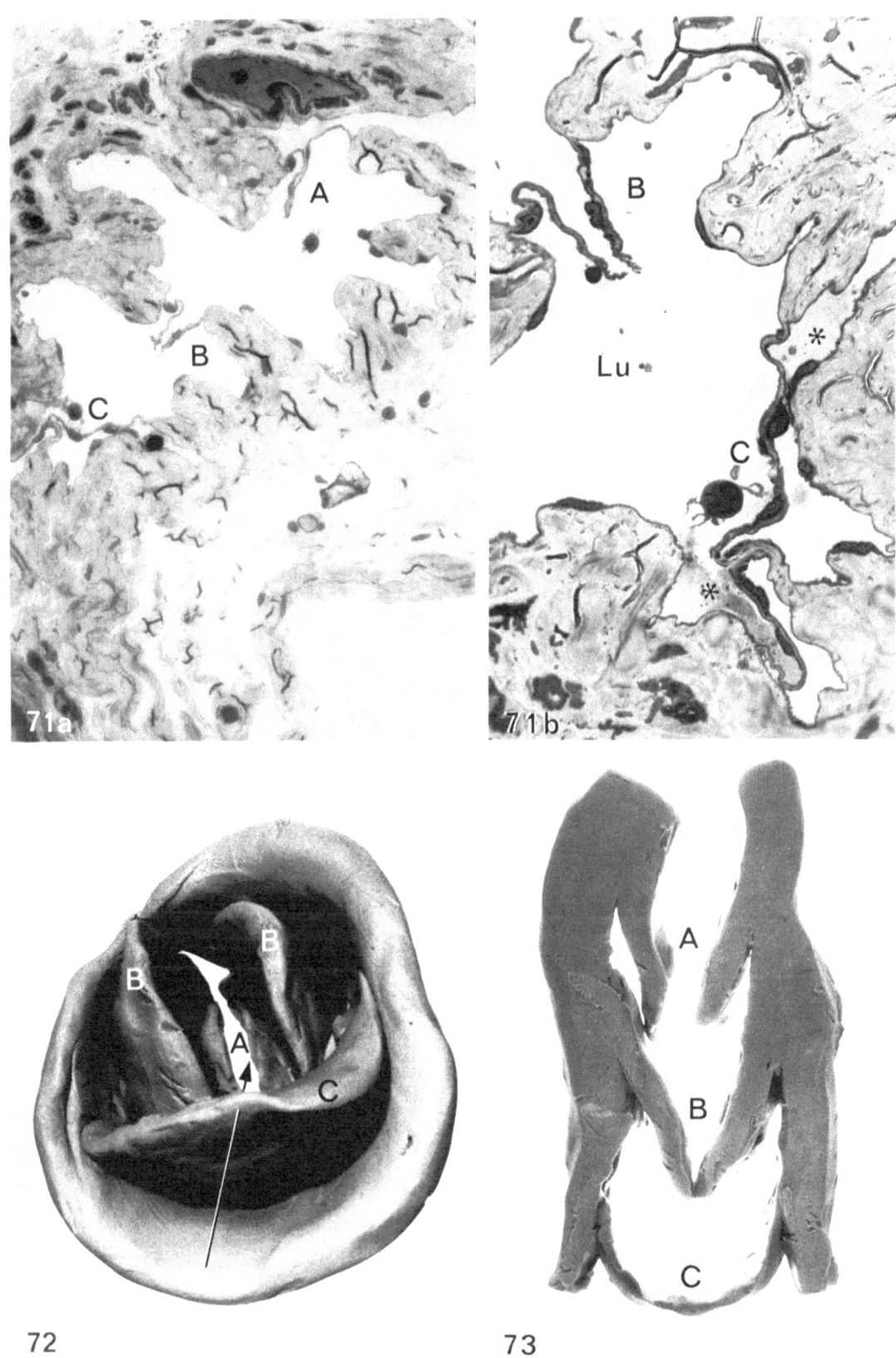

71a

71b

Lu

72   73

Fig. 74. Inflammation, eczematous rat paw skin. Bicuspid valve is seen in the dilated lymphatic capillary lumen containing erythrocytes. Four consecutive sections of the same lymphatic capillary are shown in the following figures to demonstrate the numerous ways in which valvular cusps and the modified valvular endothelial cells can appear on the sections. Semithin section; toluidine blue, × 500

Fig. 75. Section 2: The cusps of the valve are closely attached. The nuclei of the valvular endothelial cells are very prominent. × 500

Fig. 76. Section 3: The valves are accompanied by erythrocytes. The nuclei of the valvular endothelial cells are bulging into the lumen. × 500

Fig. 77. Section 4: The plane of the section arrived the tip cells protruding into the lumen *(arrow)*. × 500

Fig. 78. Section 5: Only a short compartment of the valve appears, showing endothelial cells on the luminal surface with prominent nuclei. An erythrocyte *(arrow)* is in close contact with a cytoplasmic process of the valve. × 500

Fig. 79. The cusp of the valve can be cut in this way to produce the section plane if Fig. 78

Fig. 80. This three-dimensional model demonstrates a single valvular cusp and the suggested cutting plane for reconstructing the conditions of Figs. 78 and 79

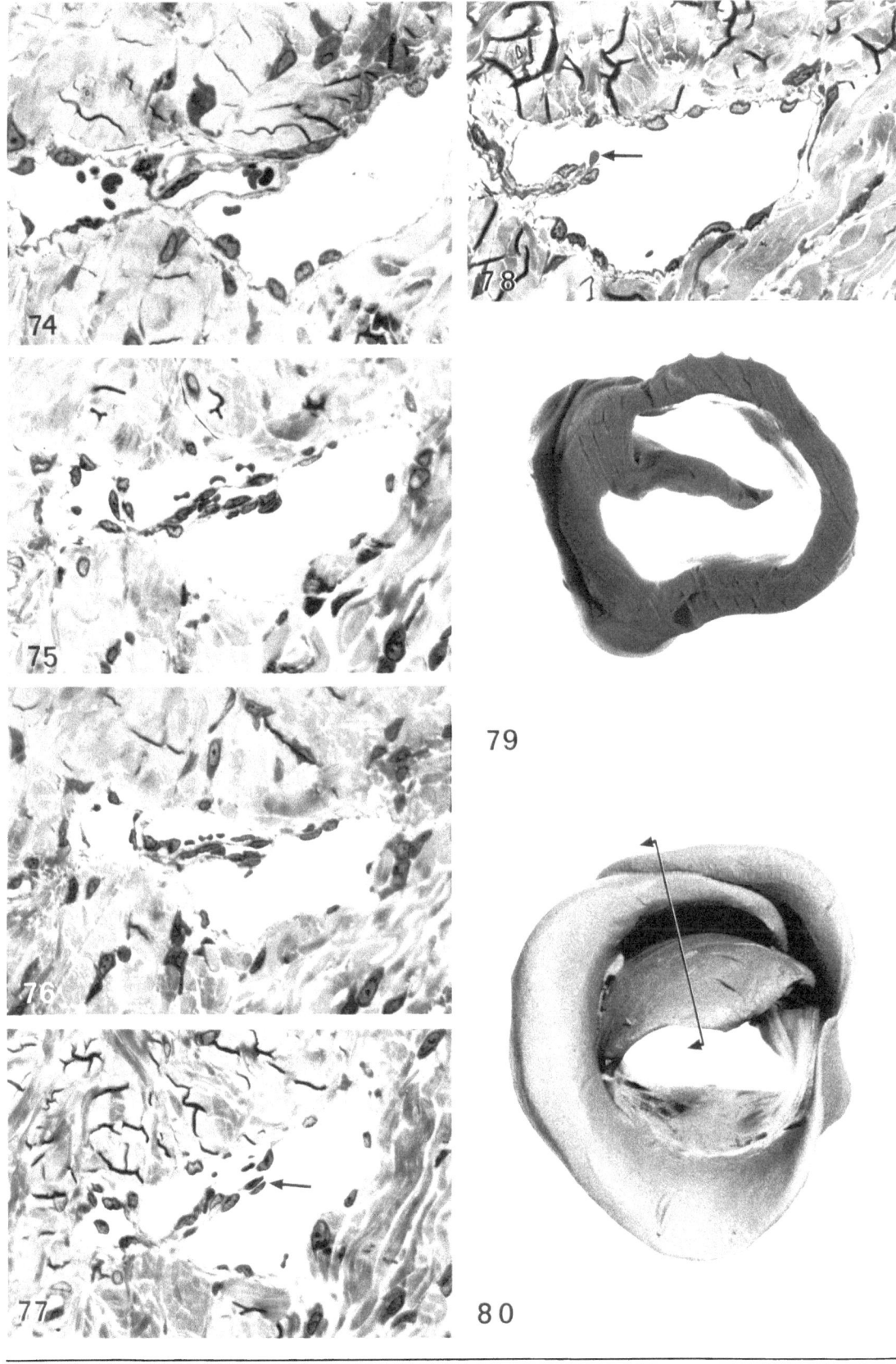

Fig. 81. Human material, ichthyosis, back skin. The endothelial cell of the lymphatic capillary has numerous contacts with the adjacent endothelial cells *(arrows)*. It spans the lumen to approach the endothelium *(End)* of the opposite side. The nulceus of this unicellular valve is indented and the cytoplasm is rich in microfilaments *(mf)*. In some places the perilymphatic basal lamina *(Bl)* is well developed. × 2500

Fig. 82. Human material, ichthyosis, back skin. Close-up of the cytoplasm of the unicellular valve that contains large numbers of microfilaments. The longitudinal and cross sections of the microfilamentous bundles *(mf)* are surrounded by mitochondria *(Mi)* and endoplasmic reticulum *(Er)*. × 16000

Fig. 83. Human material, ichthyosis, back skin. Close-up of the lymphatic endothelial cell expanding into the capillary lumen *(Lu)*. The cytoplasm contains mitochondria *(Mi)*, short tubules of endoplasmic reticulum *(Er)*, and abundant microfilaments *(mf)* 6–9 nm in diameter. × 20000

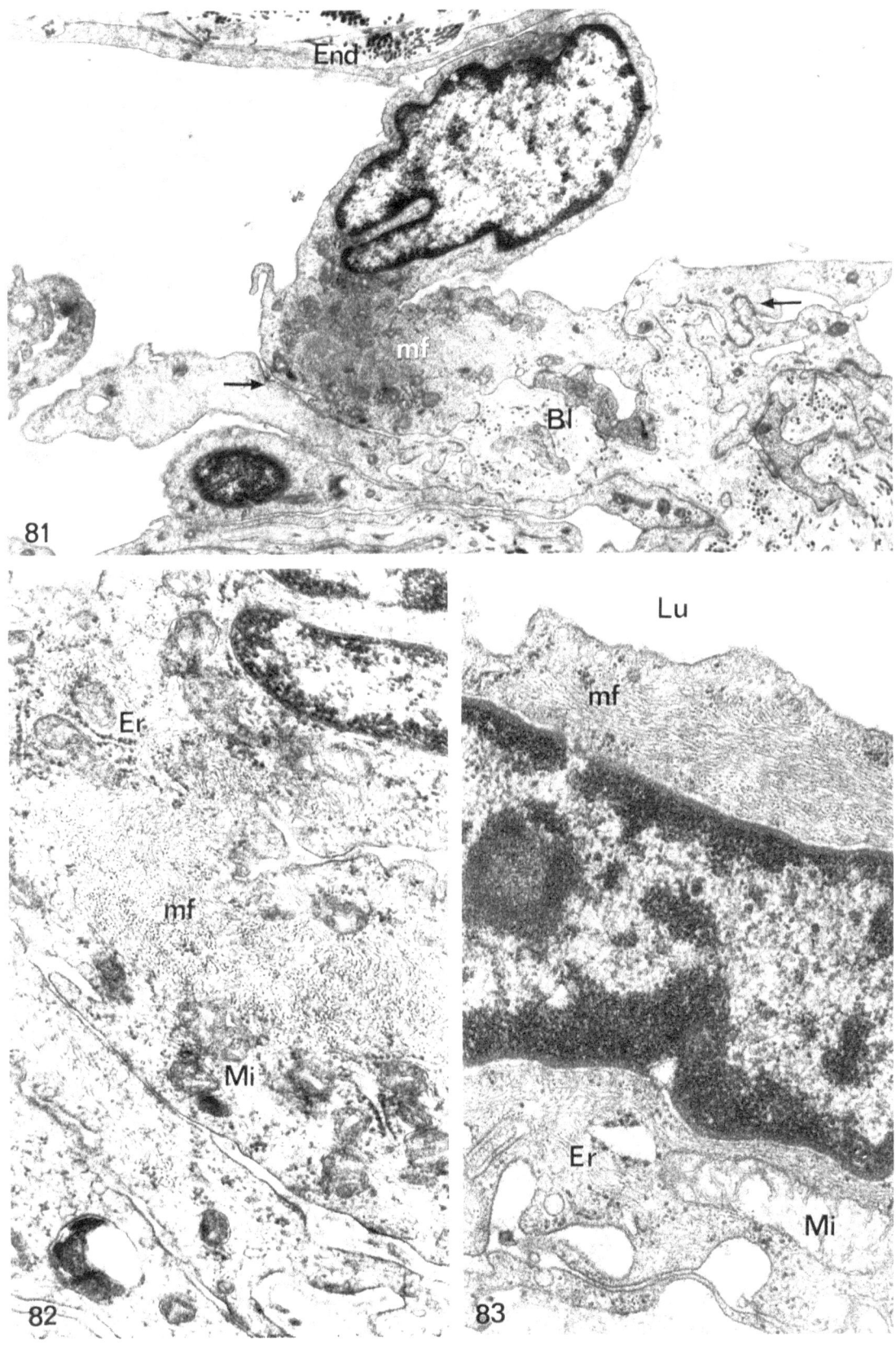

Fig. 84. Human material, pityriasis rubra pilaris, back skin. Lymphatic capillary with a unicellular valve *(arrowhead)* and a "bunch valve". The stem of the bunch consists of connective tissue folds covered by endothelial cells. Along its free edge the tip cells bud into the lumen. Semithin section; toluidine blue, × 800

Fig. 85. Human material, pityriasis rubra pilaris, back skin. Bunch valve with tip cells along the free edge of the connective tissue core. The prominent oval nuclei occupy the whole cytoplasm, extending into the lumen with narrow processes. Numerous dense attachment plates are developed between the connective tissue core and the tip cells of the lymphatic valve. × 3000

Fig. 86. Human material, pityriasis rubra pilaris, back skin. One tip cell is shown from the free edge of a lymphatic bunch valve. The surface of the modified endothelial cell displays numerous vesicles; its cytoplasm contains bundles of microfilaments *(mf)* measuring 6–8 nm in diameter. A dense attachment plate *(arrow)* is seen between two tip cells. Magn.: × 6000

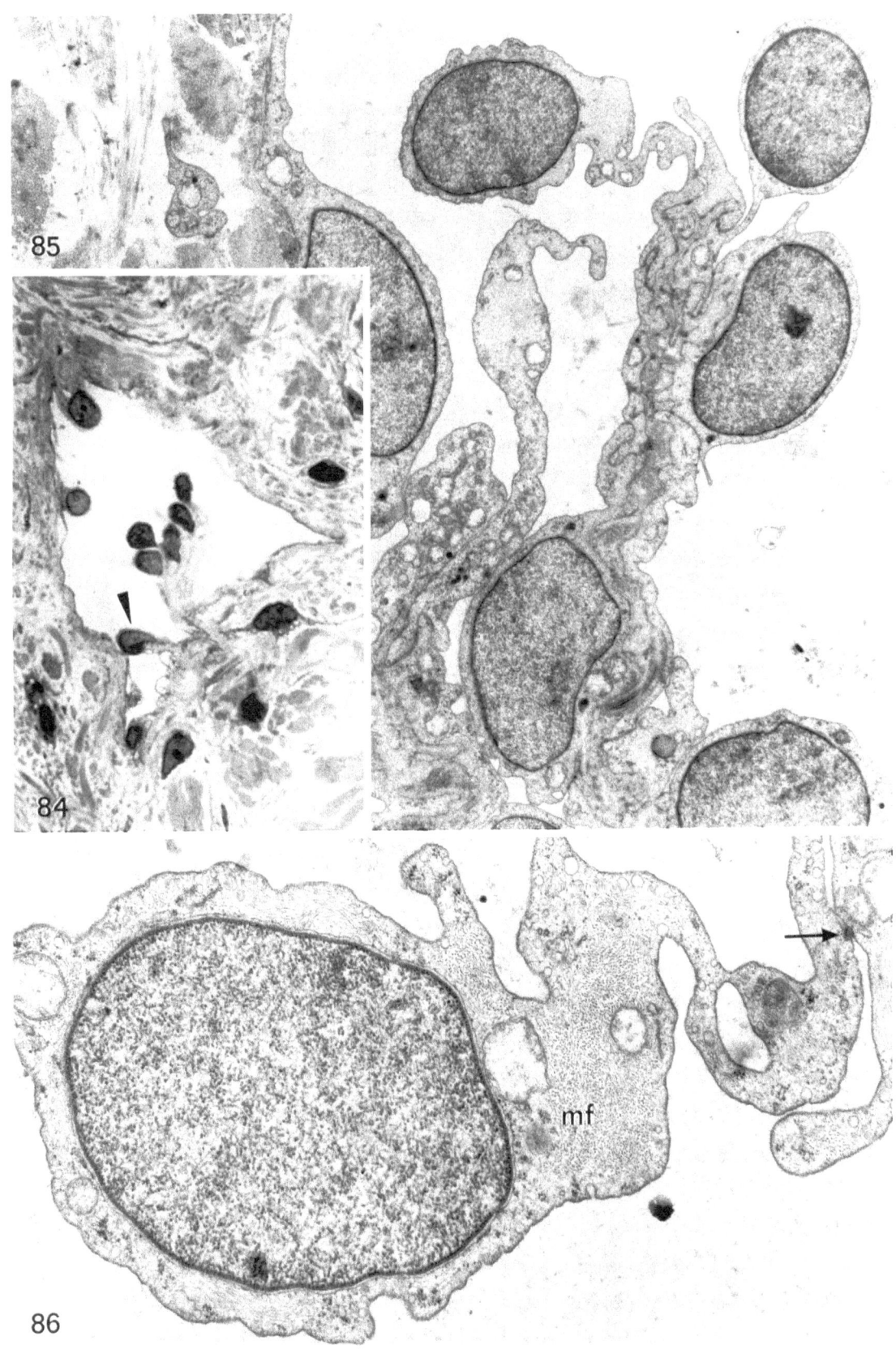

Fig. 87. The three-dimensional model shows a partly closed lymphatic capillary segment with a gap between the flaps of two adjacent endothelial cells. Planes I, II and III indicate the sections shown in Fig. 88

Fig. 88. The cut surfaces of the model shown in Fig. 87 demonstrate the advantage of serial sections in the interpretation of the real conditions of the lymphatic capillary

Fig. 89. Three-dimensional model of the site where a smaller lymph capillary *(A)* joins a larger lymph vessel *(B)*. The *arrows* indicate the section plane of Figs. 90 and 91

Fig. 90. Eczematous rat paw skin. The cut surface of the model in Fig. 89 demonstrates the "lumen-in-lumen" appearance of the joining lymph capillary. The joining capillary seems to float in the lumen of the larger vessel, as modeled in Fig. 91. Semithin section; toluidine blue, × 500

Fig. 91. This model represents the cut surfaces of the model demonstrated in Fig. 89. The smaller capillary *(A)* seems to float in the lumen of the larger vessel *(B)*, producing a "lumen-in-lumen" appearance vessel

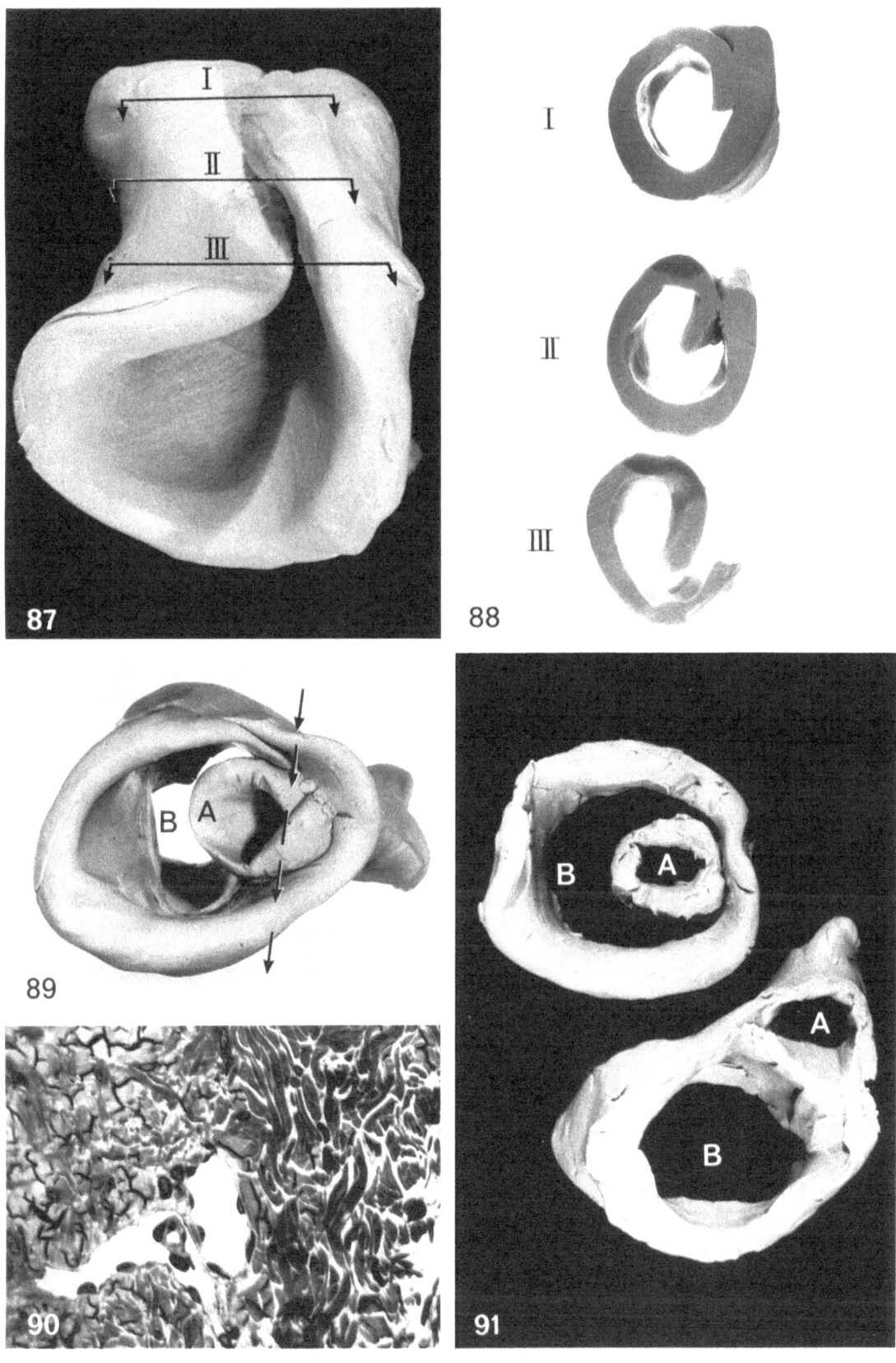

Fig. 92. Inflammation, eczematous rat paw skin. The perivascular space is directly connected with a part of the lumen *(stars)* that is surrounded by elongated processes of the endothelial cells. The other parts of the lumen, varying in size, are encircled by endothelial cell processes. The continuous basal lamina is missing and the elastic fiber *(E)* seems to be in close contact with the thornlike processes of the endothelium. × 12000

Fig. 93. Inflammation, eczematous rat paw skin. Overlapping endothelial cells of the lymph capillary close the lumen *(Lu)*. A continuous basal lamina is missing; the collagen fibers, varying in diameter, are intermingled among the increased amount of granulofilamentous ground substance. *g,* Dense cytoplasmic granule; × 10000

Fig. 94. Another section from the lymph capillary seen in Fig. 93 demonstrates the presence of a gap *(star)* between the endothelial cells that seemed to be overlapped on the other sections. The amount of basal lamina-like material *(Bl)* is increased, *g,* Dense cytoplasmic granule; × 10000

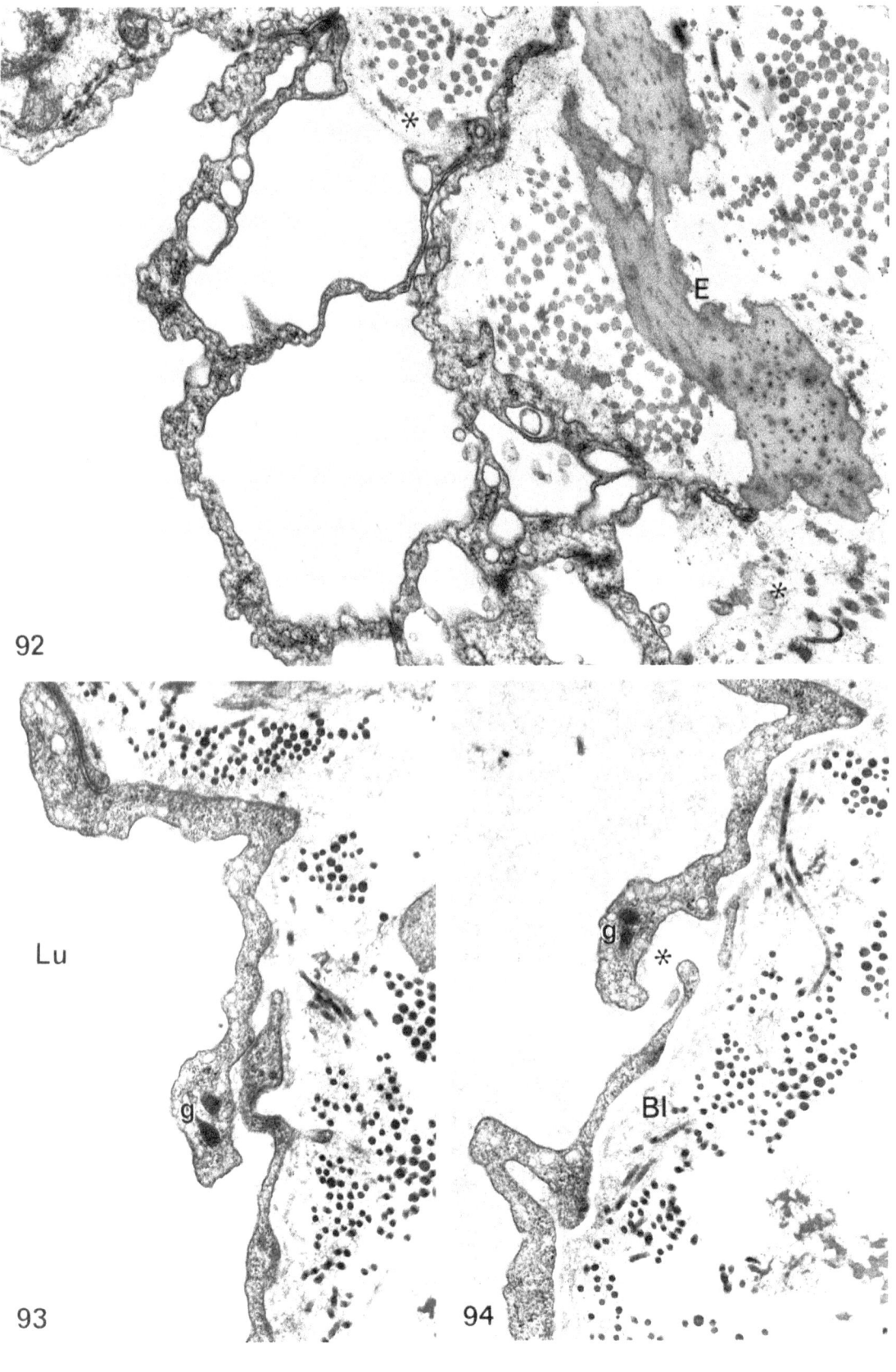

92

Lu

g

93

g

*

Bl

94

Fig. 95. Inflammation, eczematous rat paw skin. The interendothelial space and the connecting vesicles *(arrow)* with lanthanum contrast. The loose perivascular space contains microfilaments and fragments of elastic fibers *(E)*. × 14000

Fig. 96. Inflammation, eczematous rat paw skin. Unstained section showing the lumen *(Lu)* and the perivascular space of a lymphatic capillary. The particles of the native ferritin are demonstrated individually and in small groups *(thick arrows)* among the connective tissue fibers; they appear in the endothelial vesicles *(thin arrows)* and are present in the lumen. × 35000

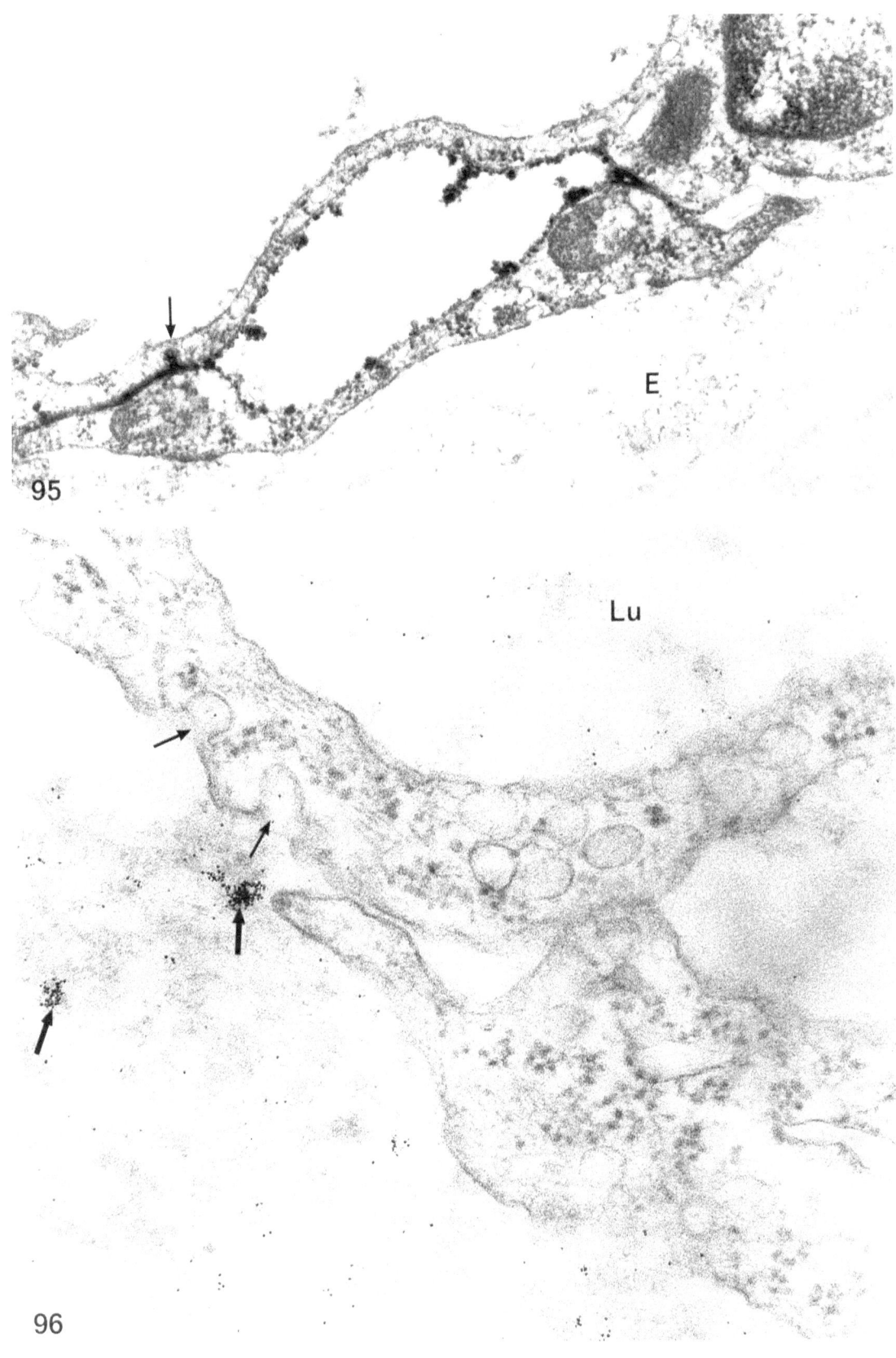

95

Lu

96

Fig. 97. Inflammation, eczematous rat paw skin. The lymphatic capillary containing erythrocytes in the lumen *(Lu)* displays a large gap in the wall *(arrow)*, producing a direct contact between the lumen and the interstitium. Lanthanum appears in large patches around the open junctions. × 5000

Fig. 98. Inflammation, eczematous rat paw skin. A connective tissue cell moving through a gap between two endothelial processes in the lymph capillary wall *(arrows)*. The extravascular process of the connective tissue cell is closely surrounded by collagen *(Co)* and elastic *(E)* fibers. *Lu,* Lymphatic lumen; × 5000

Fig. 99. Close-up of the cytoplasm of the connective tissue cell moving through the lymphatic wall shown in Fig. 98. The "neck" of the cytoplasm contains a bundle of filaments measuring 7–8 nm in diameter. The tubular connective tissue microfilaments *(f)* running directly to the abluminal cytoplasmic membrane of the endothelial cells *(End)* are in close contact with the connective tissue cells. × 20000

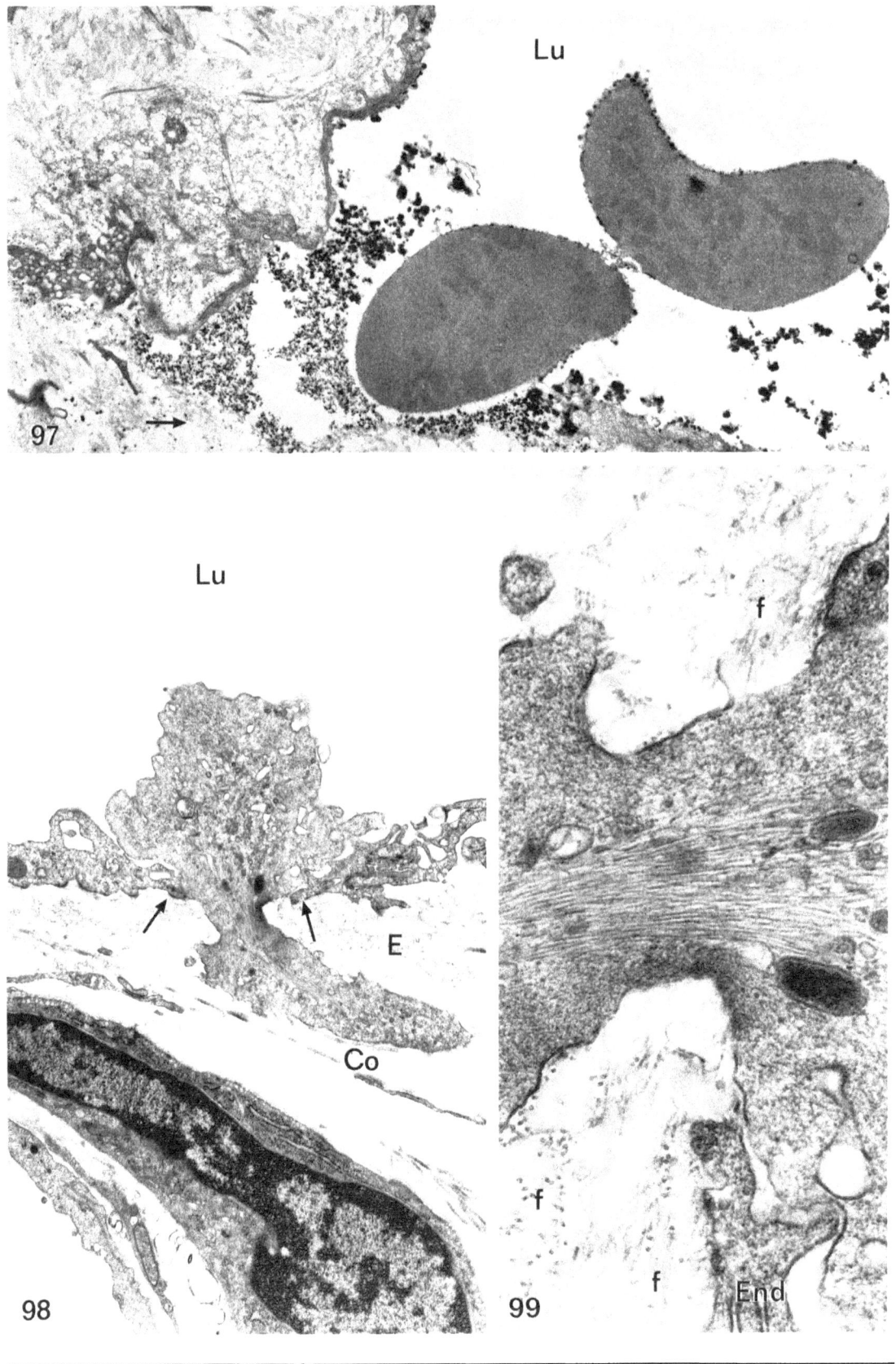

6 Lymphaticovenous Anastomoses

The term "lymphaticovenous anastomoses" is used to describe the communications between lymph vessels and veins. During embryonic differentiation, communicating vessels connect the lymphatic system to the venous system but most of these communications are lost during embryonic phase.

It is an accepted fact that in man nearly all lymph returns to the circulation by means of the thoracic duct, through its junction with the left jugular vein.

The sinusoids in lymph nodes represent a mutual lymphatic and blood chamber, being related to both blood and lymphatic vessels. Passage from the lymphatic channels to the venous system within the lymph node can occur if the intranodal pressure is elevated. Direct passage might occur when the lymphatic flow is increased, when the lymph node is squeezed, or in case of edema, efferent lymphatic blockage, infection, or tumor infiltration (THREEFOOT and KOSSOVER 1966).

Lymphaticovenous communications within lymph nodes were documented using tracers (colloidal carbon) and cells (erythrocytes and bacilli), injecting these substrates into the lymphatic system by various routes. These substances were identified in the blood, which was taken simultaneously with the injections, confirming their direct passage from the node into the circulatory system (PRESSMAN et al. 1967).

The role of the lymphaticovenous anastomoses in the spread of bacterial infections has not yet been demonstrated.

Conditions causing obstruction of the lymphatics lead to increased intralymphatic pressure, and the greater volume may be related to the development of lymphaticovenous communications. The most frequent causes for the development of lymphangiovenous anastomoses

are the blockage of lymphatic drainage by tumorous processes, surgical amputation, and removal of the lymph nodes (THREEFOOT and KOSSOVER 1966). Surgical ablatio by radical mastectomy impairs the ability of the lymphatics to transport lymph. The development of functioning lymphaticovenous communications at the axillary region may be important in preventing edema during lymphatic transport. These anastomoses are negligible under normal conditions. Iodinated (I^{125}) human serum albumin was injected intralymphatically and blood samples were taken from the vein to determine the shunting of labeled albumin. In normal volunteers and in patients suffering from severe edema after mastectomy lymphaticovenous shunting of the labeled albumin was negligible. In the non-edematous postmastectomy group the quantity of the iodinated albumin was increased.

Lymphaticovenous shunts are supposed to represent normal anatomical variations which may compensate for lymphatic destruction. The lymphaticovenous shunt can play the same role in patients with congenital defects in their lymphatic drainage (ABOUL-ENEIN et al. 1984; RUSZNYÁK et al. 1967). It is difficult to demonstrate such shunts morphologically, even with serial sections.

The most informative demonstrations of the communications between lymphatics and veins have been made with lymphangiography, using radioactive triolein and other radio-opaque media (MALEK 1972; THREEFOOT and KOSSOVER 1966). Communications were demonstrated in 52% of the cases studied. The presence of peripheral edema, malignancies, congested organs, and the administration of cardiovascular drugs were not strongly correlated to the existence of communications.

7 Lymph Formation and Lymph Flow

The fluid and protein movement and lymph formation can be described by two equations (STARLING 1896, TAYLOR et al. 1973).

The first equation relates net volume movement (J_v) to the filtration coefficient (K_{fc}) and forces acting across the capillary membrane, i.e., capillary hydrostatic pressure (P_c), tissue fluid hydrostatic pressure (P_T), and colloid osmotic pressure of plasma (π_c) and tissue (π_T). The reflection coefficient (σ_p) indicates the permeability of plasma proteins related to the capillary membrane (NICOLL and TAYLOR 1977):

$\sigma_p = 1$ if the molecule cannot permeate the capillary
$\sigma_P = 0$ if the molecule is freely permeable

Experimental evidences indicate that σ_p has a value between 0,7 and 0,95

$$J_v = K_{fc} (P_c - P_T) - \sigma_p(\pi_c - \pi_T)$$

The lymph normally forms as a result of imbalance in P_c, P_T, and σ_P ($\pi_c - _T$). The second equation described the net protein movement $= J_p$ in the transport route of the vascular bed

$$J_p = \bar{C}_p (1 - \sigma_p)J_v + PS (C_p - C_T)$$

PS = permeable surface area, $\bar{C}_p$ = average concentration difference between plasma and tissue, C_p = plasma protein concentration, C_T = tissue protein concentration.

If the lymphatics did not remove proteins from the interstitium that leaked from the capillaries then P_T would be equal with P_c which is known to be possible only in a state of severe lymphedema.

The concepts of "lymphatic overwhelming" and "lymphatic safety factor" were introduced

by GUYTON (1968) and RUSZNYÁK et al. (1967). This safety factor existing in each tissue prevents great changes in tissue hydration. They described the contribution of the lymphatics to the overall regulation of interstitial fluid volume. The change in tissue volume is the difference between the capillary volume filtration and lymph flow. Lymph flow has been shown to increase by between three- and 20-fold following an increase in venous pressure or a decrease in plasma colloids.

The long-term lymph flow safety factor is a result of growth of new lymphatics and at increases in the diameters of existing lymphatic vessels.

When the net volume movement (J_v) increases as a result of elevated capillary pressure, the tissue fluid pressure increases and tissue protein concentration can decrease. Plasma colloid osmotic pressure can increase and lymph flow can be more voluminous to oppose the increased filtration force. These compensatory changes in forces are collectively termed "the edema safety factor". Gross edema develops only after the tissue pressure becomes positive. The interstitial fluid pressure must rise from the normal value of −6.3 to above 0 before edema begins to appear. The lymph flow safety factor calculates 7 mm Hg for subcutaneous tissue. Another safety factor that helps to prevent edema is increased lymph flow. The maximally increased lymph flow gives approximately 7 mm Hg. Colloid osmotic pressure of the interstitium decreases from 4 to 1 mm Hg because of lymphoid transport of protein back to the circulation and produces a "protein-washout" safety factor of 3 mm Hg. The sum of these tissue forces (lymph flow = 7 mm Hg, interstitial fluid pressure = 7 mm Hg, protein washout = 3 mmHg) is 17 mm Hg for subcutaneous tissue. This means that the capillary pressure must rise to about 17 mm Hg above its normal value before edema begins to develop. This explains why edema develops not under normal conditions but only when severe abnormalities appear in the circulation. The safety factor can be calculated for any tissue (NICOLL and TAYLOR 1977; TAYLOR et al. 1973).

Lymph formation depends upon the production of interstitial fluid and on amounts of protein leaving the arterial capillaries, as well as upon active and passive driving forces.

The forces which normally cause tissue fluid to enter lymphatic capillaries, i.e., the mechanism of lymph accumulation, are not very well understood and the transport of the lymph in a central direction is a matter of some dispute.

The main questions one has to answer are:

1. How does interstitial fluid move across the lymphatic capillary endothelium?
2. How does lymph concentrate?
3. How is lymph transported along the lymphatic vessels toward the center?

Lymph formation depends on a suction-like action of the terminal lymphatics and on different forces which cause interstitial fluid to enter the lymphatic capillary. Starling experimentally demonstrated (RUSZNYÁK et al. 1967) the importance of plasma colloid osmotic pressure and capillary pressure as determinants of capillary filtrate and lymph flow. Basically, the average hydrostatic pressure minus the effective average osmotic pressure causes a slight volume flow into the tissue that is counterbalanced by outflow from the interstitium via the lymphatics.

It is difficult to get accurate measurements of fluids on either side of the lymphatic capillary wall. McMASTER (1946) inserted small hypodermic needles into the tissue. A small volume of fluid was then injected into the tissues and the equilibrium pressure was measured. Injury to capillaries and lymphatics along the needle possibly leads to increased local transudation of fluid and artificially elevated pressure. The technique has yielded values of +1 to −5 mm Hg for tissue pressure. GUYTON (1963) implanted perforated spherical capsules

subcutaneously and several weeks later recorded the hydrostatic pressures in the free fluid space within the capsule. This pressure was negative, averaging −6.3 mm Hg.

Pressures measured by a needle technique in plasmatic capsules implanted in tissues failed to change, in accordance with Starling's law, in experiments where the venous pressure, arterial pressure, and hydration-dehydration of the interstitium were changed.

TAYLOR et al. (1973) demonstrated that the interstitial fluid pressure is subatmospheric and that the intralymphatic pressure is positive. How can fluid move from the negative to the positive pressure system?

It is difficult to explain how lymph could be forced into tissues where the interstitial fluid pressure is negative and the pressure in the lymphatic capillaries positive. Several different forces and mechanisms are responsible for the entrance of interstitial fluid into lymphatic capillaries and for the transfer of fluid and materials.

Using improved measuring techniques in bat-wing preparations, HOGAN and NICOLL (1979) measured simultaneously the intraluminal and interstitial pressure circumstances. They found that the free interstitial pressure was greater than the intralymphatic pressure, for an average of 43% of the contractile cycle. The interstitial fluid could flow into the lymphatic along a *pressure gradient* for part of the contractile cycle. They also found that due to the pressure gradients (between luminal and interstitial pressures) during the contractile cycle the lymphatic capillary had a suction-like action on the interstitial fluid some segments away.

On contraction of the segments between two valves, called "lymphangions", the intralymphatic pressure rises above the interstitial pressure. The closing of the loose intercellular junctions and the opening of the lymphatic valves ensure the central lymph flow.

In anesthetized dogs lymphatic pressure was measured in different parts of the lymphatic system. It was concluded that the centripetal lymph flow is maintained by temporarily acting regional forces rather than by a constant pressure gradient (SZABÓ and MAGYAR 1967).

The determination of protein concentration in lymph is still quite controversal. Lymph is not identical with interstitial fluid. The lymph in the lymphatic capillaries is often more concentrated than tissue fluid (RUSZNYÁK et al. 1967).

Radioactive iodinated serum albumin was injected into mice, who were killed 24 h later. The protein in the lymph found in the lymphatic capillaries was considerably more concentrated than that in the connective tissue fluid (CASLEY-SMITH and SIMS 1976; CASLEY-SMITH 1979). The investigators envisaged an *osmotic force* sucking tissue fluid into the terminal lymphatics. Electron microscopy showed that the protein concentration of lymph in the lymphatic capillaries was about three times greater than that of the interstitial fluid. The electron density of the lumen was considerably greater than that of the tissue channels, and this density of the luminal proteins increased during the emptying phase and decreased during the filling phase (CASLEY-SMITH and SIMS 1976).

Tissue fluid therefore enters the lymphatic capillaries because of the osmotic effects of the lymph proteins. The structure of the lymphatic capillaries ensures the opening and closing of the lymphatic wall. The protein concentration in the lymphatic lumen is higher because the endothelial junctions may close during the contraction, preventing the escape of large molecules and protein. Water and small molecules are allowed to return into the interstitium.

There is some evidence demonstrating that the protein concentration in the lymphatic capillary lumen is about the same as that found in the interstitial tissue.

GUYTON (1981) described a suction-like action of the peripheral lymphatic vessels. Despite the fact that the lymphatic capillaries do not possess muscle cells in their wall, they do not lack *contractility*. The lymphatic vessels are segmented by valves. The segment between two valvular structures is called a "lymphangion" (MISLIN 1961, 1976). The occurrence of rhythmic contractions in lymphatic vessels has been described in a number of mammalian species.

Spontaneous rhythmic contractions with a frequency of 4–5/min were observed on lymphatic vessels of the human leg (SZEGVÁRI et al.

1963). Spontaneous contractions were evoked by distension of lymphatic walls. The rate of wall deformations also affected the spontaneous activity, which propagated with a velocity of 4–5 min/s (OHHASHI et al. 1980).

During lmyphangiography of the lower limbs the motility of the human lymph vessels was investigated. Contractile activity was demonstrated. The pulse appeared irregular and no specific rhythm was detected (ARMENIO et al. 1981).

The *intrinsic contractility* may be an important determinant of lymph flow. The pattern of contractility is influenced by different factors.

The lymphangions appear continuously, varying in size and shape. Variations occurred in the frequency and amplitude of contractions from segment to segment of the lymphatic chain. The lymphatics in different parts of the body show different frequencies of pulsation. The peristaltic motility and activity are provoked by an increase in internal pressure and by increased temperature of 27°–43°C (MISLIN 1961). The form of the endothelial cells is influenced by the pressure variations in the environment. This change of the stretching of the endothelial cell affects the cytoplasmic microfilaments and is presumed to cause contractions of the microfilaments. The function of the lymphatics is supported by such *extrinsic forces* as massage, muscle pump, arterial pulsation, and respiratory movements. These forces permit the entrance of fluid through the lymphatic wall. Massaging and squeezing play important roles in propelling lymph along lymphatic vessels.

The increased transmural pressure increased the strength and rate of contractions. The intrinsic pumping due to the active contractions of elements within the lymphatic wall is proposed to exert centripetal force on the lymph.

The contractile behavior of isolated guinea pig mesenteric lymphatics was studied in vitro (McHALE and RODDIE (1976), MISLIN (1961) and RODDIE et al. (1980). Increases in the rate and force of lymphatic contractions help lymph transport.

8 Function of the Dermal Lymphatic Capillaries

8.1 Functional Morphology

The lymphatics are composed of draining channels with centripetal streams of fluid traveling from peripheral tissues to the central lymphatic tunnels.

The most characteristic feature of the lymphatic capillaries is that they change their dilatation. At the relaxation stage they are collapsed, without visible lumen; the interdigitating, overlapping, wrinkling endothelial cells are indistinguishable from the connective tissue fibroblasts. Depending on the interstitial load, lymphatic capillaries dilate 10–50 times more than at rest. They change their shape and their connections and relationship to the surrounding connective tissue.

Structural properties facilitating dilatation of the dermal lymphatic capillaries are as follows:

1. A continuous basal lamina is missing, or it may be scanty or interrupted. The interstitial pressure forces (hydrostatic, osmotic pressures) may act immediately, without any structural impediment, on the capillary endothelium.
2. Pericytes are lacking; the interstitial forces may act directly on the capillary wall.
3. Special connections of the endothelial cell processes do exist: end-to-end, overlapping, interdigitating, accordion-like wrinkles. The loose connections between the neighboring wall endothelial cells allow movement of the endothelial cells over each other; they can move away from each other, they can change their shape, becoming flat from being round or oval, and the wrinkles can be flattened – the lymphatic wall straightens as the lumen dilates.

4. The tubular connective tissue microfilaments measuring 10–12 nm in diameter are directly connected with the abluminal membrane of the endothelial cells. These fibers are elastic microtubules; they can be embedded in the elastic matrix. They anchor the endothelium to the connective tissue of the perivascular space. Collagen fibers can also be connected directly with the capillary endothelial cells. The close linkage of the lymphatic capillary wall with connective tissue fibers makes possible direct transmission of interstitial pressure to lymphatic capillaries.
5. The endothelial cells contain actin-like cytoplasmic microfilaments. Dilatation of the lymphatic wall probably triggers the contraction of bundles of endothelial microfilaments.
6. The lymphatic capillaries possess valves that facilitate central lymph flow. The valve system includes inlet valves (interendothelial) and intraluminal valves.

The inlet valves are inconstant, transitory structures that develop between the neighboring endothelial cell processes along the capillary wall and respond to local pressure variations and intraluminal-interstitial pressure gradients.

The intralymphatic valves (joining, segment, unicellular, bunch valves) are able to seal the lumen, and, like "lock gates", they maintain an unidirectional (centripetal) lymph flow and develop the pumping function of the lymphatic capillaries. In response to local pressure variations, the connective tissue folds of the valves may vary in length and width. For example, in one phase rising interstitial pressure forces push the valve core deeper into the lumen, while in another phase increed intraluminal pressure pushes connective tissue folds back into the connective tissue of the wall (Schema 2).

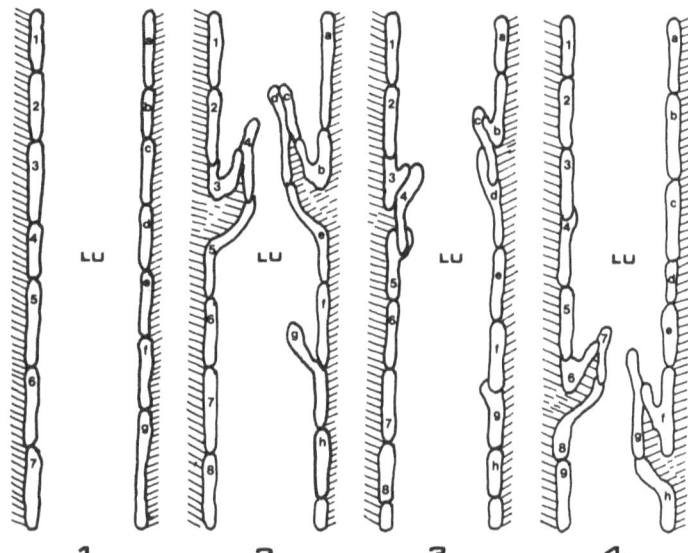

Schema 2. Four different phases of activity, the rearrangement of the wall endothelial cells, and the new formation of the valves. *1,* Capillary at rest. *2,* New valve is created due to the protruding of connective tissue and endothelial cells; *g,* unicellular valve. *3,* The temporary valve structures (connective tissue backbone and endothelial cells) are sliding back to the wall endothelial cells. *4,* New temporary valves are formed along another capillary segment

It is supposed that local pressure differences can create temporary valves. The pressure changes modify the wall endothelium by transformation into valvular endothelial and tip cells. The final shape of the valves and the tip cells probably depends on suction forces activated in the lumen which generate elongated, spindle or comma-shaped modified endothelial cells and pseudopodia.

Bunch valves and unicellular valves probably facilitate the lock-gate function of the capillary segments by acting as "flap" or "helping" valves. When the pressure wave is over these "temporary" valves slide back into the wall structures.

8.2 Manner of Function

The forces which normally cause tissue fluid to enter the lymphatic capillaries are a matter of some dispute. They are:

1. Hydrostatic pressure
2. Osmotic pressure
3. Intrinsic and extrinsic forces

In normal dermis the tissue hydrostatic pressure is negative, less than atmospheric (about −6.3 to −6.5 mm Hg), while intralymphatic pressure is approximately atmospheric.

As blood capillary pressure forces fluid and materials into the interstitium and the fluid volume increases in the interstitium, this expands the interstitial space, and the collagen and elastic fibers move apart due to the high tension. The tension is transformed to the lymphatic capillary wall by the inserted microfilaments; therefore, the endothelial wall is pulled open by the connective tissue filaments (CASLEY-SMITH 1967; LEAK 1976).

Stretching of the wall trigger contraction of the cytoplasmic actin-like filaments. Their contraction enhances the development of the interendothelial junctions. The overlapping of the adjacent endothelial cells serves as a reserve supply of the capillary wall that can be utilized for rapid dilatation.

The interstitial fluid pressure in local areas rises temporarily to a positive value and causes the overlapping endothelial processes to open. The less – than – normal negative pressure in the interstitium allows the interstitial fluid to enter into the lymphatic capillaries. The cellular processes open and close as a one-way flap-valve system.

When the intraluminal pressure is equal to or higher than the interstitial pressure the flap valve is closed. This results in the widening of the lumen and the opening of the patent junctions. The injection of hyaluronidase into the foot pads of rats caused the lymphatics to collapse. This was presumably the result of a solubilization of connective tissue ground substance and a disruption of anchoring filaments (CASLEY-SMITH (1967; LEAK 1972a).

The concept that the interstitial fluid flows from the tissue spaces into the lymphatic capillaries along a pressure gradient has gained the support of direct experimental evidence from bat-wing preparations (HOGAN and NICOLL 1979, ZWEIFACH 1973).

The rapid passage of fluid and materials from the interstitium into the lymphatic lumen is permitted by these intercellular junctions. The vesicular route through the cytoplasm serves as an important but slower passageway. The interendothelial patent junctions are open during tissue relaxation and the filling phase, and they are closed during tissue compression and the emptying phase. Lymph flow into the lymphatic capillaries is favored by the osmotic pressure difference between the interstitium and intraluminal lymph.

The protein concentration of the lymph in the lymphatic capillaries is higher than that in the connective tissue fluid. This indicates that the lymphatic capillaries concentrate the fluid they receive from the perivascular space (CASLEY-SMITH and SIMS 1976).

The lymph flow into the lymphatic capillaries is enhanced by extrinsic forces such as arterial pulsation, respiratory movement, and massage of the connective tissue and by intrinsic forces such as contraction of actin-like cytoplasmic filaments, causing increasing stretching of the wall. These forces cause the opening of inlet valves, which permits to the entrance of fluid and material into the lymphatic capillaries. Schema 3 of the dermal lymphatic capillaries.

At rest the tissue hydrostatic pressure (THP) is negative (about -6.3 mm Hg) and the intraluminal pressure (LHP) is atmospheric. As blood capillary pressure forces fluid into the interstitium the THP rises and temporarily (along a given section) becomes higher than the LHP, thereby generating a hydrostatic pressure gradient from the interstitial space to the lymphatic capillaries.

The increased fluid pressure within the interstitial space expands the connective tissue components. The collagen and elastic fibers are moved apart pulling, the capillary wall with which they are connected. The stretching of the wall induces active contractions of the endothelial cells. The pressure differences force the inlet valves to open, and fluid and large molecules enter and dilate the lymphatic lumen. This is the "filling" phase. The lymph will be dilated. As rising intraluminal pressure closes the inlet valves, the black-flow of the lymph is prevented.

Central lymph flow from one segment to the next lymphangion is favored both by hydrostatic and colloid osmotic pressure differences between the distal and proximal lymphangions and by the intrinsic contractility of the lymphangion itself.

During the next stage proximal intralymphatic valves open and distal valves are forced to close, propelling the lymph into the proximal lymphangion. The intramural interendothelial junctions are closed, preventing the escape of the proteins and other large molecules into the interstitium. Only some fluid can regurgitate into the interstitial space through cytoplasmic pores. Proteins and other macromolecules, however, are retained in the lumen. Thus, lymph flowing centrally is continuously concentrated. This is the "emptying" phase.

In the maintenance of central lymph flow temporary and regional forces such as endothelial valve structures probably play an important role. The segments of the lymphatic capillaries with inlet and intraluminal valves probably work as tiny pumps. The periodic pumping and suction of the lymphatic capillaries propels lymph into the larger lymphatic channels, which exert a suction effect.

The lymphangions can contract independently of one another. The dermal lymphatic capillary network constantly remodels itself in

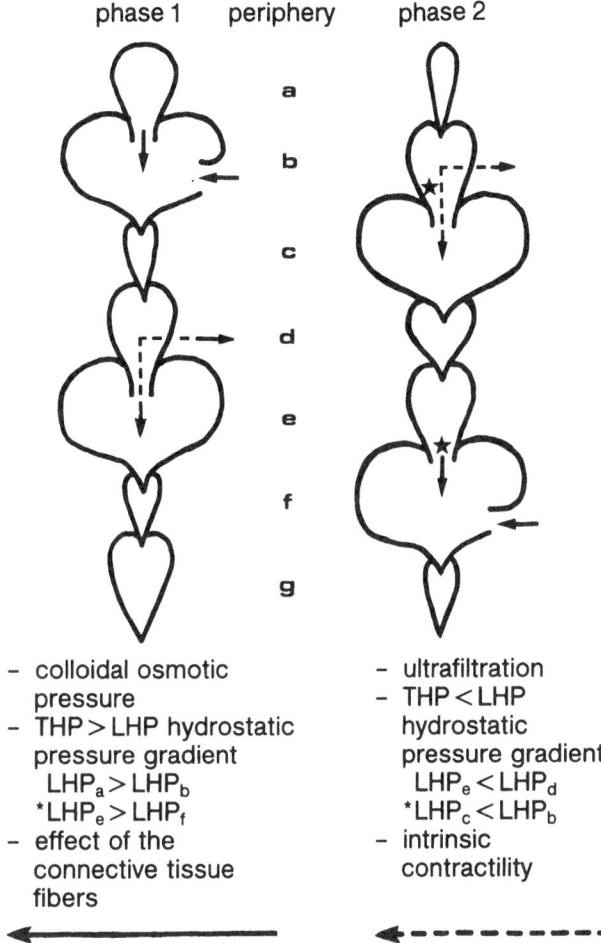

phase 1   periphery   phase 2

- colloidal osmotic
  pressure
- THP > LHP hydrostatic
  pressure gradient
  $LHP_a > LHP_b$
  $*LHP_e > LHP_f$
- effect of the
  connective tissue
  fibers

- ultrafiltration
- THP < LHP
  hydrostatic
  pressure gradient
  $LHP_e < LHP_d$
  $*LHP_c < LHP_b$
- intrinsic
  contractility

Schema 3. The piston function of two identical regions of a lymphatic capillary lymphangions a–g. The solid *arrow* represents the forces hydrostatic pressure gradient, osmotic pressure gradient, effect of connective tissue fibers causing the fluid to enter into the capillary lumen and/or to flow further into a proximal lymphangion. The *dotted arrow* indicates the forces causing the lymph to leave the capillary lumen and/or to flow into a proximal lymphangion (ultrafiltration, intrinsic contractility, hydrostatic pressure gradient)

response to interstitial conditions (inflammation, edema). Finally, the shape of the lymphatic valves varies considerably and depends largely on endothelium-connective tissue interactions. The third schematic drawing illustrates the pumping and suction forces operating during the filling and emptying phases. Identical segments demonstrate the postulated *piston function.*

Hydrostatic and osmotic pressures force the interstitial fluid into the lymphatic lumen (lymphangions b and e) while at the same time suction forces favor the movement of the lymph from the distal lymphangions (lymphangions a and d) centrally. These forces operate simultaneously in variable phases. The alternating pumping and suction phases of lymphatic capillary function resemble those of a piston.

9 The Role of Interstitial Proteolysis and Macrophages

The absence of lymphatic capillaries from different tissues (brain, bone marrow, retina, superficial endometrium) has been shown in various species. This absence produces the problem of the clearance of interstitial proteins and fluid in these tissues (LAUWERYNS and CORNILLIE 1984).

The role of cellular activity has been extremely neglected in the analysis of the fate of extravascular interstitial plasma proteins. Macrophages play an important role in the clearance of the interstitium. Plasma proteins escaping from the blood circulation become phagocytosed and are stored and catabolized in the tissues by macrophages or undergo extracellular proteolysis.

LAUWERYNS and CORNILLIE (1984) have reported results of their study on protein clearance from rat endometrium using colloidal ferritin and carbon as protein tracers. Large pleomorphic phagocyes were present in the perivascular interstitium. These interstitial phagocytes accumulated large amounts of lipofuscin and hemosiderin. Numerous monocytes leaving the circulation developed pseudopodia and differentiated into active phagocytes, engulfing interstitial substances by means of cytoplasmic vacuoles.

The ferritin and carbon particles were phagocytosed by macrophages. The tracer particles never appeared to accumulate in interstitial tissue channels or prelymphatics.

Interstitial monocytes internalize and digest interstitial proteins. The intracellular lipid droplets indicate the high proteolytic activity of the phagocytes. Proteolysis reduces the colloid osmotic pressure in the interstitium. It is postulated that protein molecules of reduced molecular weight or the smaller segments of large molecules may drain via the fenestrations of the venous blood capillaries. Our study also demonstrated fenestrated capillaries in the papillary dermis and around the skin appendages (DARÓCZY and HÜTTNER 1978).

The venous drainage of protein and fluid is important in these regions. Interstitial proteolysis is an alternative clearance mechanism in tissues lacking lymphatic capillaries.

10 Pharmacology of the Dermal Lymphatic Capillaries

The function of the dermal lymphatics can be modified by influencing the permeability, the motility, and the contractions of the vessels. The rhythmical contractions are of major importance for the propulsion of lymph.

The increased interstitial pressure is indirectly adequate to provoke contractions of the capillary wall. The extrinsic (contraction of muscles, pulsation of arteries) and intrinsic factors (contraction of actin-like cytoplasmic filaments of the endothelial cells) can be influenced directly by mediators and drugs. Drugs can affect the lymph flow by:

▷ Changing the effective filtration pressure of the arterial capillaries
▷ Changing the venous pressure
▷ Changing the permeability of the capillaries
▷ Promoting the breakdown of the protein molecules of the interstitial fluid
▷ Altering the stretch of the lymphatic endothelial wall: stretching of the wall causes the contractions of the actin-like microfilaments; i.e., the motoric activity of the lymphatic capillaries will be affected.

It is concluded that mediators and drugs affect the hemodynamics and the permeability of the blood-capillary barrier.

Considering the threshold concentration of the drugs studied (noradrenalin, serotonin, histamine), the lymphatics react less sensitively than do arteries and veins.

Studies investigating the influence of biochemical mediators and drugs on lymphatic motility deal mostly with isolated lymphatic vessel preparations. The main objects of these studies are the mesenteric and thoracic lymphatic vessels.

Positive and negative chronotropic as well as positive and negative ionotropic effects can be registered, depending on the species, the part of the body from which the portion of vessel derives, and also the vascular segment actually being investigated (LEHMANN 1983). The amplitude and the power of the contractions depend on the concentrations of the drugs.

Increased blood flow was observed parallel with the increase of lymph flow brought about by histamine (VOGEL 1972). ATP, ADP, and cyclic AMP lead to relaxation of the mesenteric lymphatics. Epinephrine increases the rate of contraction but reduces the strength of the individual contractions. The effect is dose dependent. In high doses a fibrillation of the perilymphatic muscle cells was observed.

Isoproterenol reduces the rate of contraction but causes some increase in the strength of the individual contractions. In high doses it causes suppression of thoracic duct activity. In the mesenteric vessels it leads to relaxation.

Acetylcholine increases the lymph flow in both the thoracic duct and the limbs, leading to a higher filtration volume into the interstitium. Papaverine increases the lymph flow by causing reduced arterial resistance (RODDIE et al. 1980). In a low concentration, bradykinin accelerated the rhythm of contractions in bovine mesenteric lymphatics (AZUMA et al. 1983).

The vasomotor effects of norepinephrine, serotonin, isoproterenol, and histamine in vitro can be abolished by specific antagonists. Phenylbutazone abolishes the increased lymph flow induced by bradykinin but does not antagonize the increased lymph flow following papaverine administration (LEHMANN 1983).

These observations suggest that bradykinin increases the permeability, whereas hemodynamic factors are of no significance for its pharmacodynamic action.

Prostaglandins are detectable in human lymph under inflammatory conditions. The ability of the human dermal lymphatic vessels to generate prostacyclin in significant amounts has been described (MANNHEIMER et al. 1980), but its role is not yet quite clear. Prostacyclin, or $PG1_2$, is a derivative of arachidonic acid and caused reductions (in a concentration of $10^{-6}\,M$) in the amplitude of spontaneous contractions. Prostaglandins (PGF_{2alfa}, PGA_a, and PGB_a) in low concentrations may facilitate lymph flow (bovine mesenteric lymphatics), causing increases in the frequency and amplitude of spontaneous contractions in isolated bovine mesenteric lymphatics (JOHNSTON and GORDON 1981; OHHASHI and AZUMA 1984).

The contractions induced by prostaglandins are not inhibited by antihistamines, serotonin antagonists, or alfa- or beta adrenergic blocking agents. The spontaneous contractions could be inhibited by aspirin (cyclooxygenase inhibitor) and by inhibitors of thromboxane synthetase (JOHNSTON and GORDON 1981).

CASLEY-SMITH et al. (1969) successfully treated lymphedema with pantothenic acid and pyridoxine. The mechanism of action was suggested to be a quick breakdown of the interstitial protein molecules.

Calcium ions are important for controlling the propagation of the impulse and the contractile response. Isolated bovine mesenteric lymphatics were studied in different calcium concentrations. Reduction of the Ca^{2+} concentration decreased the amplitude of spontaneous contractions; increased external Ca^{2+} decreased the frequency of the spontaneous contractions and finally stopped them (AZUMA et al. 1983; McHALE and ALLEN 1983).

It is not clear what is the in vivo significance of the findings obtained in isolated lymphatics or how dermal lymphatics react under physiological conditions. Some observations on the effect of epinephrine and histamine on the dorsal surface of the human foot have been made. SZEGVÁRI et al. (1964) demonstrated that the lymphatics increased their activity under the influence of epinephrine and histamine. Changes in the activity of lymphatic smooth muscle affect the propulsion of the lymph. Biochemical mediators act presumably on the lymphatic muscle cells; their isometric tensions and action potentials were investigated on isolated mesenteric lymphatics.

The direct actions of the mediators on the dermal lymphatic capillaries (having no smooth muscle cells in their walls) are not yet understood. Mediators and drugs can affect the transport and composition of the interstitial fluid.

A direct effect of histamine, bradykinin, and prostaglandins on lymphatic motility cannot be excluded. The pharmacology of the lymphatics remains a neglected field. Practically speaking, the direct pharmacological control of dermal lymphatic function is not known.

11 Inflammatory Conditions

11.1 Morphological Changes of the Dermal Lymphatic Capillaries During Inflammation

Lymphedema is a form of inflammation. Excessive accumulation of fluid and proteins can be observed in chronic inflammation due to vasodilatation and disorganization of the vascular endothelial wall.

Thermal injury, resembling acute inflammation, was produced (50°–60 °C) in animal experiments (CASLEY-SMITH 1973b; LEAK 1972a), and the main morphological findings were summarized as follows: Morphological changes observed in lesins occurring at 50 °C were decreased electron opacity of the endothelial cells due to the swelling of the cytoplasm, an increased number of cytoplasmic vesicles, dilated endoplasmic reticulum, and swollen mitochondria. The changes were developed and very striking in 3-h lesions but conditions returned to normal by 48 h. The alterations produced by 54 °C injury were more severe: numerous open junctions between the endothelial cells and disorganization of the cytoplasmic microfilaments. These changes were transient and showed signs of reversal 12 h after heat injury. The elastic microtubules anchoring the epidermis to the connective tissue were revealed after injury at 50°–54 °C.

Thermal injury at 60 °C produced severe degenerative changes of the lymphatic capillaries. Open endothelial gaps, dilated capillary lumina, and activated endothelial cells provide an increased lymphatic capacity in inflammation.

As long as the safety-valve function of the activated lymphatics is not exhausted, the increased lymphatic load can be propelled through the lymphatic vessels.

11.2 Regeneration of the Lymphatic Capillaries

The regenerative capacity of the dermal lymphatic vessels is enormous. The rapid regeneration of the small vessels in the skin graft was demonstrated by microangiography.

After degenerative processes the reactive proliferation of new lymphatic capillaries is very quick and can supply the regenerated region. The newly regenerated lymphatics are sensitive to radiation. Traumatic alteration or obliteration of the lymphatic capillaries is rapidly compensated by the opening of collaterals leading to the functioning adjacent lymphatics.

11.3 Cellular Components in the Capillary Lumen and in the Pericapillary Space

Some cells migrate through the blood vessel into the interstitial tissue and then into the lymphatics. From the connective tissue large molecules, cells, and bacteria must be transported via the lymphatics. The peripheral lymph may contain only a few cells which under normal conditions can occasionally be seen. There are neutrophil leukocytes, monocytes, lymphocytes, erythrocytes, and Langerhans' cells. In peripheral lymph collected from leg lymphatics more than 80% of the cells were lymphocytes (SOKOLOWSKI et al. 1978).

In inflammatory conditions (eczema, edema) fibrin thrombi can be revealed in the lymphatic capillary lumen (Fig. 100). The fibrin masses are usually located along the endothelial pseudopodia protruding into the lumen and valvular cusps.

Lymph clots in 10–20 min, while blood clots in 4–8 min; the interplay with platelets and fibrinogen is missing. The skin lymphatics have a negligible prothrombin content. Plasminogen is 40% of that in plasma. The antiplasmin level is only 27% of the plasma level. In filariasis, coagulation is an important cause of lymphatic obstruction.

Neutrophilic leukocytes taking active part in the inflammatory processes are most often seen in a degranulated condition. The size and the contrast of the membrane-bound lysosomes depend on the digested substances. Some cytoplasmic granules varying in density can be discovered extracellularly, floating in the lumen (Fig. 101).

Erythrocytes can be found in the connective tissue in different conditions produced by different causes, such as mechanical injury or infection. The erythrocytes can enter into the lymphatic lumen from the connective tissue area, but it is very probable that temporary shunts can be created between the venous and lymphatic dermal capillaries. For a long time the lack of erythrocytes in the capillary lumen was taken as a morphological sign of the lymphatic nature of the capillary under study. In the electron-microscopical era of lymphatic research it has become evident that erythrocytes can be detected in capillaries whose morphological features identify them as lymphatic capillaries (Fig. 102).

In lymph obtained from a patient with lymphedema after lymph node excision the levels of IgG and IgA were found to be low, whereas the IgM level was high. All complement components, as well as the C_3 level, proved to be low (OLSZEWSKI 1977). Bacteria discovered in lymphatic capillaries of rat paw dermis showed intact membranous structures and vacuolated cytoplasm (Fig. 103).

Macrophages have not been a rare finding in the lymphatic capillary lumina of inflamed or edematous skin. The surface of such macrophages was characterized by elongated cytoplasmic processes. In some cases they seemed to float freely in the lumen, but in other capillaries the cytoplasmic pseudopodia seemed to be pushed to the luminal surface of the capillary endothelium. Circulating macrophages have a large amount of cytoplasm containing cisternae of endoplasmic reticulum, polyribosomes, well-developed Golgi complexes, dense granules, centrioles, and mitochondria. The nucleus may be round, oval, or indented (Figs. 104–107).

Some reports suggest the interstitial accumulation of mast cells, eosinophilic leukocytes, and basophils in filarial lymphedema. The release of histamine and humoral vasoactive substances from the degranulating mastocytes and basophils increases the permeability of blood capillaries and the rate of lymph formation. The result would be a local accumulation of protein-rich interstitial fluid (i. e., lymphedema; COLVER and RYAN 1983; DUMONT et al. 1983; OTTESEN et al. 1979; RUSZNYÁK et al. 1967).

Mastocytes presenting elongated pseudopodia have been found frequently in lymphedematous human skin. The mastocytic granules with the typical laminated crystalloid morphological patterns varied in size and density, and some huge irregular granules contained lipid droplets (Fig. 108).

Dermal fibroblasts and histiocytes demonstrate high activity. These cells are rich in cytoplasmic organelles. They have well-developed Golgi complexes, and the dilated endoplasmic cisternae are full of granular material (Fig. 109).

In the huge dermal macrophages intracytoplasmic collagen fibers can be seen. The membrane-enveloped collagen fragments show a specific longitudinal periodicity of 65–70 nm (Fig. 110). Collagen phagocytosis by the dermal macrophages that digest the pathologic collagen fibers is one of the clearance mechanisms which are activated in edemic processes.

Besides the numerous macrophages, the dermal infiltrate consists of lymphocytes, plasma cells, and fibroblasts (Fig. 111). Occasionally Langerhans' cells can also be observed. The dendritic Langerhans' cells marked by tennis-racket-shaped granules with a crystalloid internal structure are usually surrounded by lymphocytes (Fig. 112). The interstitial macrophages appearing in close vicinity to the lymphatic capillary contain lipid droplets, dense pigment granules, and siderosomes (Figs. 113 and 114).

Melanin pigment can be phagocytosed by macrophages due to the degeneration of apoptotic epidermal keratinocytes. The apoptosis of the basal epidermal cells represents a possibility for eliminating damaged keratinocytes. In edema epidermal keratinocytes can be damaged by being stretched over the swollen dermis or by the presence of inflammatory epidermotropic cell infiltration.

The dense siderosomes phagocytosed by the macrophages are developed due to the degeneration of the extravasated erythrocytes. In edema, the lymphatic endothelial cells can also contain dense granules in their cytoplasmic phagosomes (Fig. 115).

11.4 Role of the Lymphatic Capillaries in the Development of Cellular Immunity

Lymphatics are required to convey antigen, together with macrophages and Langerhans' cells, to lymph nodes for lymphocytic recognition. The lymphatic vessels direct the antigen from the epidermis to the lymph nodes. Without lymphatics cellular immunity could not develop.

In the case of allogenic skin grafts, the major transfer route of antigens to the lymph node is along the lymphatic pathways. Removal of the lymph drainage channels caused temporary cessation of the cellular reactions of the lymph nodes, until lymphatic pathways were re-established (LAMBERT et al. 1965).

Intact lymph drainage is indispensable for the sensibilization of the host against the grafted skin. Interruption of the lymph drainage obstructs the afferent limb of the immunological reflex circle and therefore delays rejection (BARKER and BILLINGHAM 1968; HUTH 1983).

The concentration of IgG and IgM in normal lymph measured after Mancini's radial immunodiffusion technique was about 50% of that in serum. The complement activity was very low, being 5%–11% that of the serum. In edemic limbs of dogs the lymphocytotoxic titer of the lymph was very low with respect to the total complement activity. This fact may explain the recurrence of infections in limbs with lymph stasis.

The cytolytic activity of the lymph for bacteria and foreign cells might be limited as well (OLSZEWSKI 1977). The white cell count in the peripheral dermal lymphatics seems to be low under normal conditions and increased during inflammation.

Fig. 100. Inflammation, eczematous rat paw skin. Fibrin masses *(star)* are seen in the lymphatic capillary lumen *(Lu)*. The basal lamina *(Bl)* is partially thick. The neighboring vessels *(V)* are blood capillaries. × 3200

Fig. 101. Normal human skin, lower leg. A neutrophilic leukocyte *(Leu)* in the lymphatic capillary lumen *(Lu)*. Specific granules *(g)* and lysosomes *(star)* are seen in the cytoplasm and some cell remnants are found extracellularly *(arrow)*. The elastic fibers *(E)* are in contact with the endothelial cells. × 4800

Fig. 102. Inflammation, eczematous rat paw skin. Erythrocytes *(stars)* are seen in the lymphatic capillary lumen, in which the elongated valves are floating *(arrows)*. × 2000

Fig. 103. Inflammation, eczematous rat paw skin. Detail of a dermal lymphatic capillary with a bacterium in the lumen *(Lu)*. × 3200 *Inset:* Close-up of the bacterium in the lymphatic lumen. × 10000

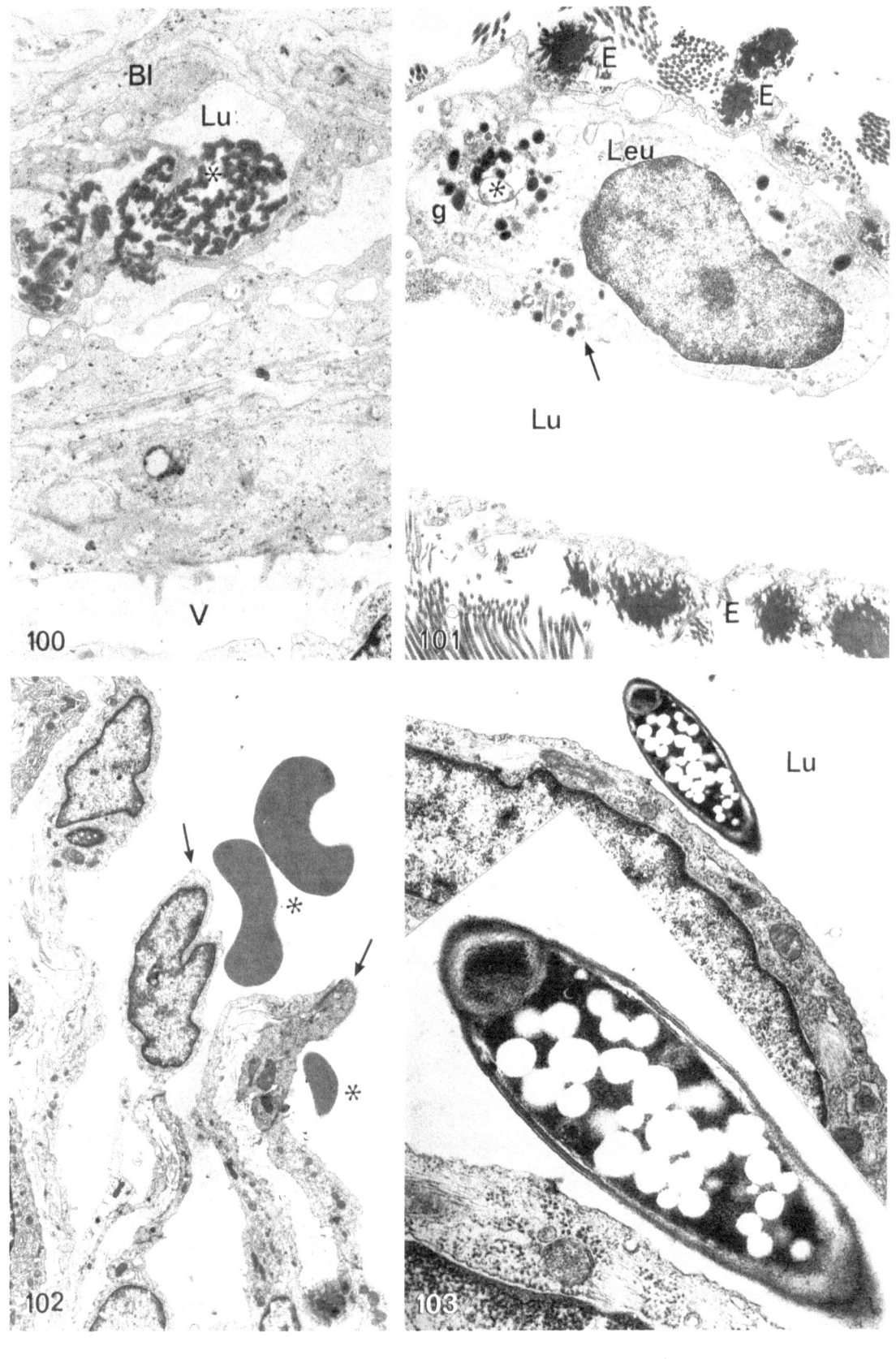

Fig. 104. Toxicoderma, human skin, upper arm. The lumen of the dermal lymphatic capillary *(Lu)* is almost filled with a large mononuclear cell that displays a very active cytoplasm, showing labyrinth-like tubules of endoplasmic reticulum *(Er)*, mitochondria *(Mi)*, and centrioles *(Ce)*. The perilymphatic space is occupied by a loose network of microfilaments and collagen fibers *(Co)*. × 5500

Fig. 105. Inflammation, eczematous rat paw skin. Overlapping, interdigitating, and open cellular junctions *(arrow)* are found in the cellular wall of the lymphatic capillary. The surface of the intraluminal cell is characterized by pseudopodia *(p)*. × 5000

Fig. 106. The whole intraluminal macrophage of which a part is seen in Fig. 105. The "hairy" appearance of the surface is due to the numerous slim pseudopodia. × 5000

Fig. 107. Lymphedema, human lower leg. The elongated pseudopodia of the intralymphatic macrophage are convoluted *(stars)* because the cell seems to be pushed to the endothelial wall *(End)*. × 5000

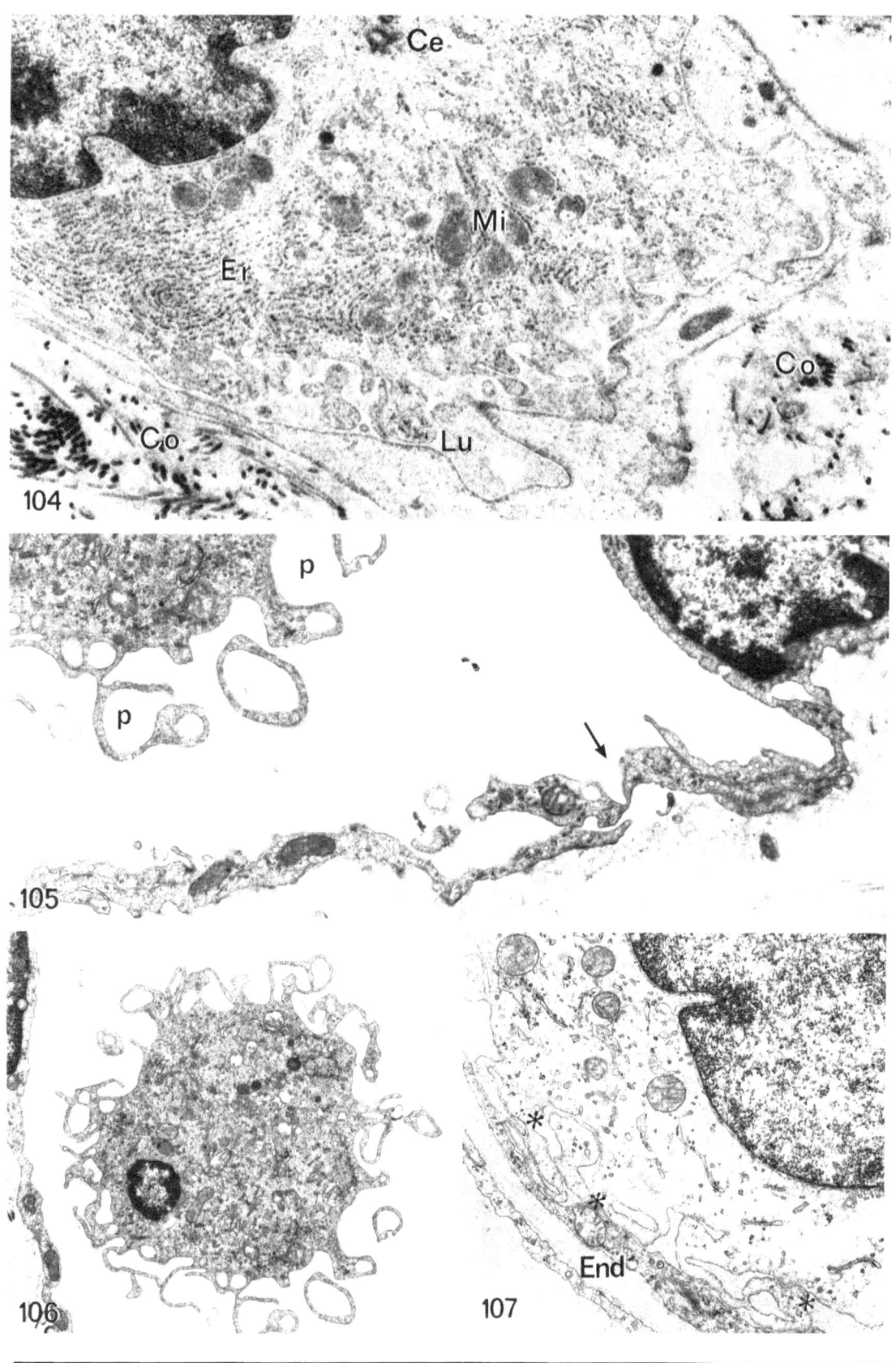

Fig. 108. Lymphedema, human lower leg. Detail of a mastocyte from the cell infiltrate of the perilymphatic interstitium. Besides the typical lamellar mastocyte granules, atypical variants are observed. In the large granule lipid droplets are embedded in the lamellar substructure *(arrow)*. × 8400

Fig. 109. Lymphedema, human lower leg. Detail of a plasma cell from the interstitial cell population. The dilated cisternae of the endoplasmic reticulum *(Er)* are filled with dense fine granular material. × 4800

Fig. 110. Lymphedema, human lower leg. Detail of connective tissue macrophage *(Ma)*. In the cytoplasm numerous intracellular fragments of collagen fibers *(arrows)* are discovered. If the intracytoplasmic segment is longer, the typical longitudinal periodicity can be demonstrated *(Co)*. The inclusions are partially membrane bound. × 7200

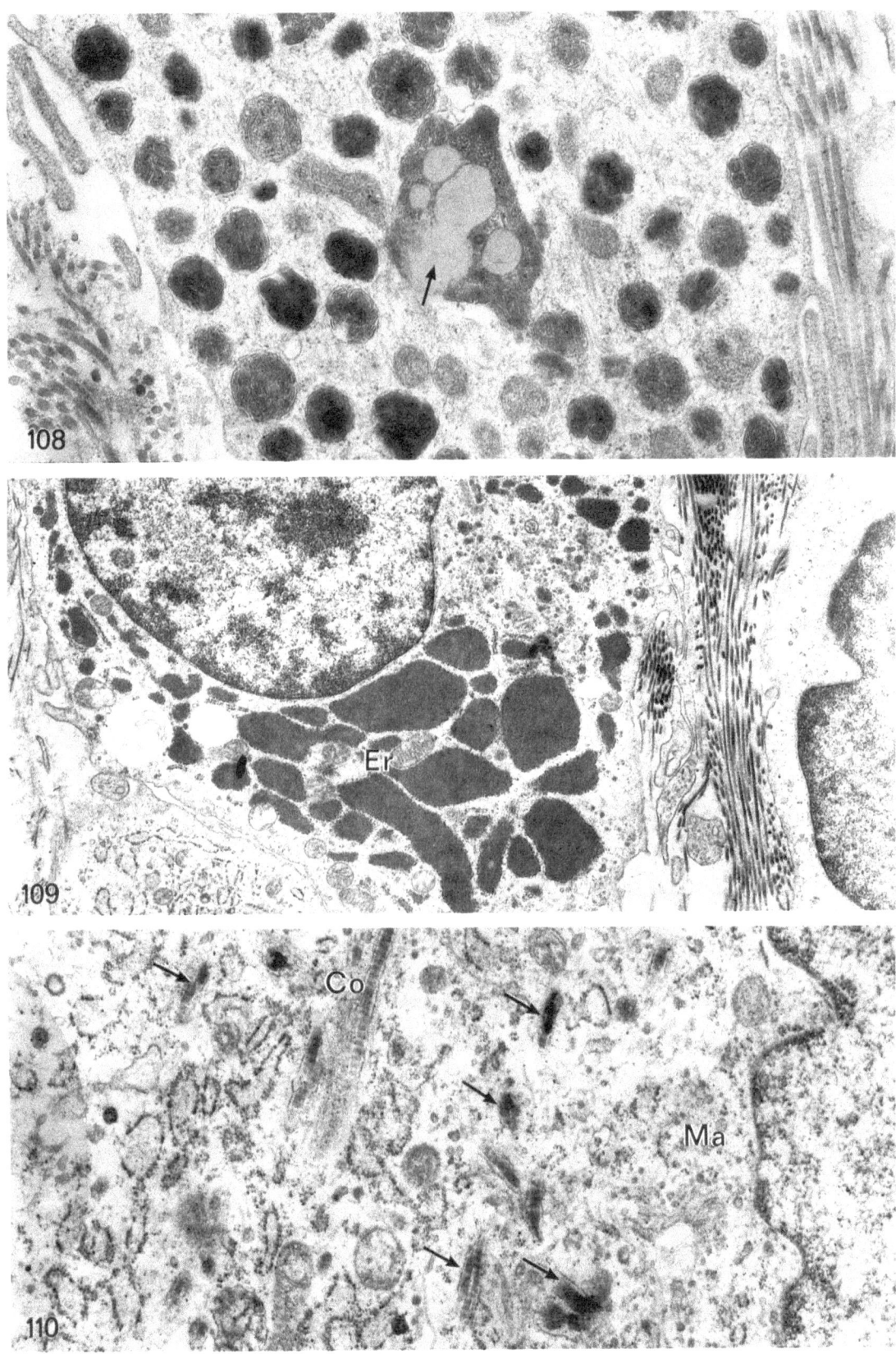

Fig. 111. Lymphedema, human lower leg. A mixed cellular infiltrate is seen in the edemic interstitium around a small dermal venular capillary *(V)*. *P,* Plasma cell: *ly,* lymphocyte; *Ma,* macrophage; *F,* fibroblast; × 10000

Fig. 112. Circumscribed lymphangioma, human skin, chest wall. Detail of dermal Langerhans' cell with the typical cytoplasmic granules *(arrows)* and a lymphocyte *(ly)* are shown from the perilymphatic mild infiltration. × 13000 *Inset:* Close-up of the tennis-racket-shaped forming Langerhans' granules *(arrows).* × 30000

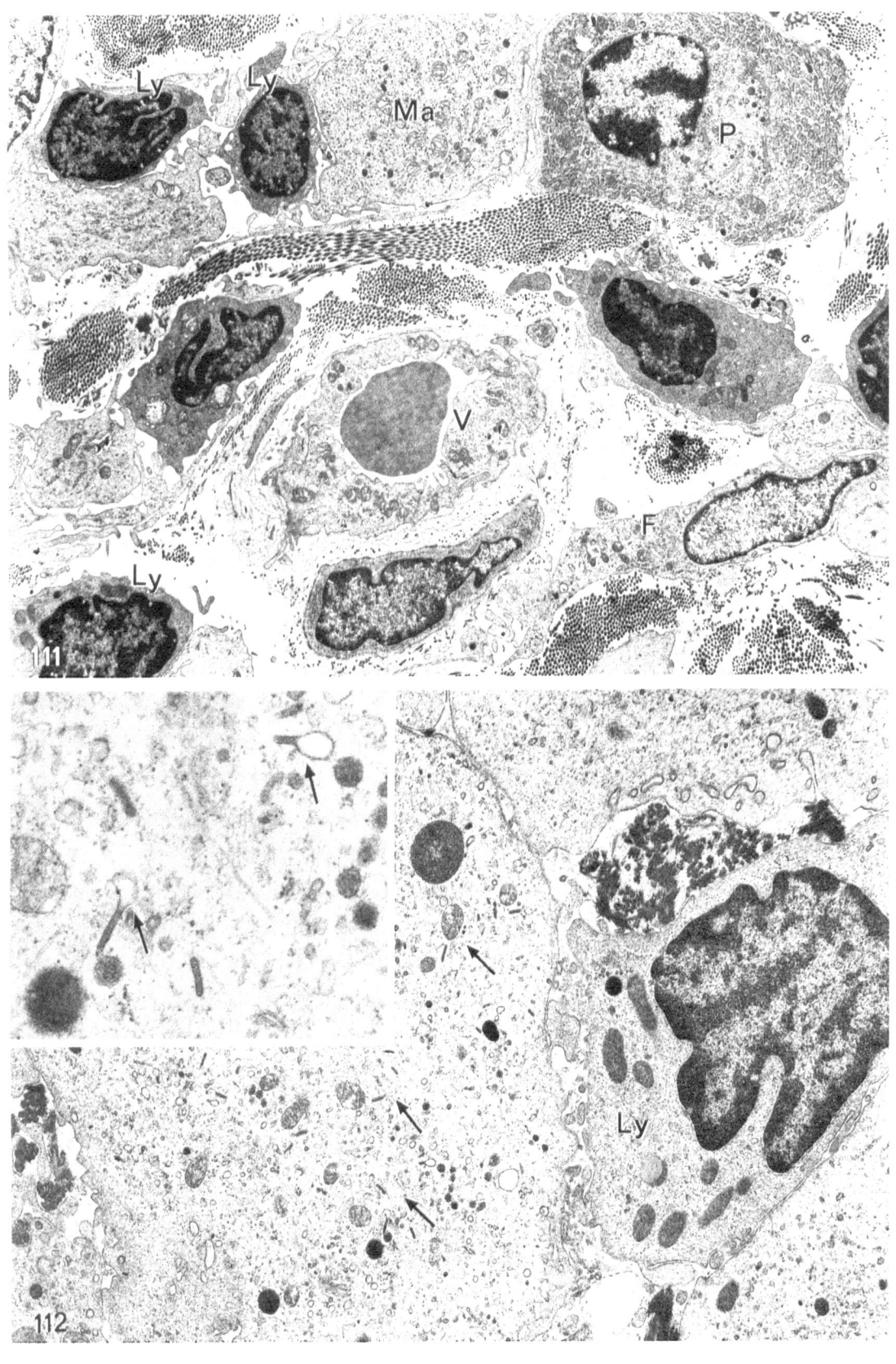

Fig. 113. Inflammation, eczematous rat paw skin. Cytoplasmic detail of a connective tissue macrophage *(Ma)* in the perilymphatic space. The phagosomes *(arrows)* are very dense. *Lu,* Lymphatic lumen; × 12000

Fig. 114. Lymphedema, human lower leg. Around the dilated lymphatic capillaries *(L)* the connective tissue macrophages are loaded with lipid droplets and pigment granules that are partially remnants of melanin pigment, partially siderosomes. × 5000

Fig. 115. Lymphedema, human lower leg. The lymphatic capillary endothelial cells contain dense membrane-bound phagosomes *(arrows)* that may be siderosomes. The perilymphatic elastic fibers *(E)* are partially fragmented and degenerated *(star). Lu,* Lymphatic lumen; × 10600

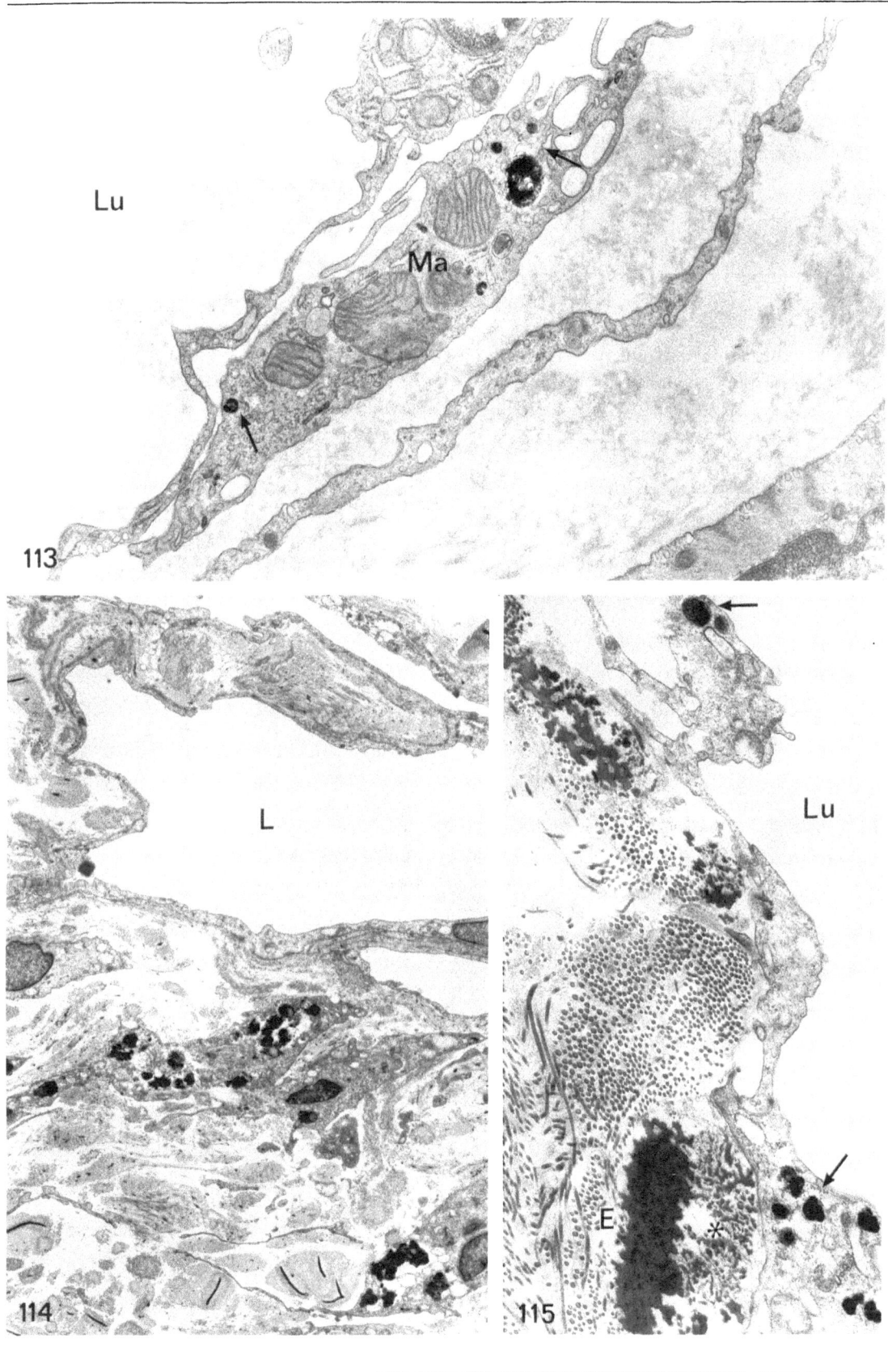

12 Mechanism of Transport
Through the Lymphatic Capillary Wall

Excess interstitial fluid and proteins are transported by the lymphatic capillaries, but there is some controversy about the mechanism of transport through the lymphatic endothelium. The main possibilities under discussion are:

1. Transport by intracytoplasmic vesicles
2. Passage between adjacent endothelial cells
3. Diffusion through the cytoplasm

All these pathways do exist, and they vary with the functional activity and with the local conditions of the lymphatic capillaries. The pathway through the capillary endothelium depends on the molecular weight and diameter of the transported material and on the species studied. Many other factors influence the selective permeability of the capillary endothelium (CASLEY-SMITH 1964 a).

Reaction products of horseradish peroxidase have been used as electron-opaque tracers to follow this protein across the blood-tissue-lymph interface. Within 1 min peroxidase staining is observed along the blood endothelial plasma membrane within the lymphatic lumen. The reaction product reaches its maximal concentration between 15 and 30 min; thereafter its intensity declines suddenly, so that by 24 h very little staining is observed (LEAK 1971).

Some peroxidase staining occurred in pinocytotic vesicles, with a greater concentration within the cleft of intercellular junctions. These observations suggest that the *intercellular junction* is the *major channel* for rapid passage of fluid and large molecules, while *vesicular transport* is perhaps responsible for the slow transendothelial passage of large molecules (LEAK 1972a). The number and the volume density of

the cytoplasmic vesicles increased after the tracer injection. Both coated and uncoated small and large vesicles could be identified in increased numbers after tracer injection (YANG et al. 1981). Peroxidase staining is also observed in phagosomes of the interstitial macrophages.

Tracer studies, using tracers of different diameters such as ferritin or colloid carbon, have established that by increased fluid/protein movement *fluid and* large *molecules pass* from the connective tissue into lymphatic capillaries, *mainly through the gaps of intercellular endothelial junctions* (CASLEY-SMITH 1965; LEAK 1971; O'MORCHOE et al. 1980; YANG et al. 1981). The endothelial junctions open either because of the pulling activity of the connective tissue filaments or as a consequence of the pressure gradient between the extracellular space and the lymphatic lumen. DOBBINS and ROLLINS (1970) found that in transendothelial transport (observed in the intestinal villi of mice and guinea pigs) the endothelial vesicles were more involved than the intercellular junctions.

Open junctions are considered to play only a small role in lymph formation under normal conditions, but they are important in conditions where there is increased fluid movement, such as inflammation, injury, or increased blood vessel permeability. Vesicular transport plays an important role in the translymphatic protein movement, but it accounts for only a small portion of the substances which traverse the lymphatic endothelium under normal conditions. Cytoplasmic transport is more voluminous in lymphedema: lipid droplets and phagosomes are numerous in the endothelial cells under edematous conditions (see Figs. 42 and 43).

13 Insufficiency of Lymph Flow

13.1 Safety-Valve Function of Lymph Flow

If the vascular filtration is increased the lymphatic system can also increase its capacity and can propel much larger amounts of protein and fluid than in the normal resting condition.

The increased lymphatic load is accompanied by an increased lymphatic transport capacity. This is the safety-valve function of the lymphatic system that prevents edema formation as long as the lymphatic transport capacity is not exhausted (Földi 1969; Taylor et al. 1973).

13.2 Dynamic Insufficiency (High Lymph-Flow Failure)

Dynamic insufficiency of the lymph flow will occur if the equilibrium between the lymphatic load and the transport capacity of the lymphatic system is disturbed. There is a close relationship between blood vessels and lymphatics in controlling tissue homeostasis. Small molecules and fluids leave the connective tissue predominantly via venules. However, large molecules and cells are too large to re-enter the venous capillaries. These substances must be removed via the lymphatics.

The *lymphatic load* is the amount of plasma protein in the capillary filtrate which cannot leave the connective tissue through the venous capillaries.

The *transport capacity* of the lymphatic system is the product of the total cross section of the lymph vessel system and the lymphatic forces (intrinsic lymphatic contraction, extrinsic factors, function of valves, pulsation of arteries). When the balance between lymphatic load and lymphatic transport capacity is upset,

the increased lymph load exceeds the lymphatic transport capacity: the tissue colloid osmotic pressure is raised; fluid remains in the interstitium, retained by high osmotic pressure of the tissue proteins – high lymph-flow failure is produced. Venous and lymphatic processes can lead to chronic edema: the chronic venous hypertension increases the blood capillary pressure; this leads to the disturbance of Starling's equilibrium, and the capillary filtration is increased. The consequence is chronic edema with dynamic insufficiency of lymph circulation, accompanied by increased intralymphatic pressure and resulting in chronic lymph block (Clodins 1977).

13.3 Mechanical Insufficiency (Low Lymph-Flow Failure)

When the equilibrium between the lymphatic load and the transport capacity of the lymphatic system is disturbed in that the lymphatic transport capacity is reduced below the level of the normal lymphatic load, low lymph-flow failure is produced.

13.4 Safety-Valve Insufficiency

In acute dermal inflammation the lymphatic safety-valve function drains the excess lymphatic load, proteins, cellular debris, and fluid and reduces the consequences of the inflammation. If acute inflammation occurs in a dermal region characterized by low lymph-flow failure, massive edema and tissue necrosis are the consequences.

Safety-valve insufficiency of the lmyph drainage occurs if low lymph-flow failure is combined with an increased lymphatic load.

14 Forms of Lymphedema

Among the various classes of edema the most important differences are whether the protein concentration in the tissue fluid is low or high and whether in high protein concentration the flow of fluid through the tissues and lymphatic channels is rapid or slow. The low protein concentration type of edema appears when the excess fluid leaving the blood capillaries cannot be transported by the lymphatic system, e.g., due to raised venous pressure or hypoproteinemia. The high protein concentration type of edema appears when a trauma of the blood vessel wall causes excessive amounts of protein and fluid to enter into the tissues, because of caused by injury to the arteries or burns, for example.

High-protein-concentration, low-flow edema is also called lymphedema, but several authors use this term to describe the swelling of soft tissues. To avoid any misunderstanding, the term "lymphostatic edema" would be more appropriate than "lymphedema" (FÖLDI 1983).

The above-mentined forms of edema can be mixed, and in these cases the interpretation of the chronic lymphedema is difficult.

14.1 Classification of Lymphostatic Edema

Primary lymphedema may develop due to malformation of lymph vessels – aplasia, hypoplasia, or hyperplasia, congenital or non-congenital. In some cases the abnormality of the vessels cannot be detected by lymphangiography because the lesions are localized in the capillaries that are not visible with this method.

Secondary lymphedema may develop for different reasons and by different mechanisms, e.g., inflammation (in lymphangitis or rheuma-

toid arthritis) trauma, tumorous involvement of lymph nodes, surgical dissection of the lymphatics, resection of the lymph nodes with or without irradiation, paralysis, muscle disorders. Various clinical types of obstructive lymphedema have the same clinical, radiological, and biochemical consequence. Not all patients, however, develop lymphostatic edema (the swollen arm or limb syndromes) after the different events that can lead – with high incidence – to the development of lymphedema.

Some factors are thought to prevent or to compensate for lymphedema:

1. Collateral lymph circulation
2. Regeneration of the lymph vessels
3. Lymphaticovenous anastomoses
4. The phagocytic system – the macrophages – digesting the proteins. The fragmented protein may leave the interstitium via venular fenestrae, and the lymph block is bypassed in this way.

14.2 Clinical and Morphological Stages of Lymphostatic Edema

There are several clinical stages of lymphedema: latent edema (early stage), manifest edema (reversible and irreversible), and elephantiasis.

14.2.1 Latent Edema

In the early stage the lymphedema disappears during the resting period (overnight). In this stage the differential diagnosis from venous edema is difficult. The edema is pitting; secondary tissue alterations are not yet present.

With lymphangiography, mural insufficiency is demonstrable, with extravasation of the contrast medium that remains in the perivascular spaces.

In some cases, latent lymphedema does not progress to the manifest stage until provoked by accidental trauma, infection, or artificial injury (lymphangiography).

Histologically, the lymphatic vessels are dilated; they display numerous open junctions and the thin valve structures are relatively insufficient. The collagen fibers are swollen and separated by the interstitial fluid. Some mononuclear cells are seen around the lymphatic and blood vessels.

14.2.2 Manifest Edema (Reversible)

Recurrent episodes of limb edema resulting in pitting edema of the dermis characterize this stage. The swollen skin is pale, and the dermis can not be picked up in folds on the dorsal aspect of the toes and fingers (STEMMER's sign). Stemmer's sign is negative in venous edema (STEMMER 1976).

With lymphangiography, the contrast medium is extravasated due to severe lymphatic hypertension accompanied by mural insufficiency of the lymphatic capillaries. The mural insufficiency involves both the capillaries and the collecting lymphatics (SOLTI et al. 1971). Histologically, the numerous lake-like channels of the dermal lymphatic vessels are surrounded by increased amounts of metachromatic ground substance. The collagen bundles are increased in relative volume and the elastic fibers are diminished in the upper and mid dermis. The elastic fibers are randomly arranged around the dermal lymphatics. The macrophages and lymphocytes are increased in number and dispersed among the connective tissue fibers.

14.2.3 Manifest Edema (Irreversible)

In this stage of lymphedema the secondary tissue changes are very prominent; the edema is non-pitting. Histologically, the lymphatic capillaries and the collecting vessels are dilated. Some intercellular junctions are permanently open, as the valve structures are insufficient. The basal lamina can be folded several times around the lymphatic capillaries. Macrophages, lymphocytes, and fibroblasts can be revealed in the perivascular infiltrate. The protein accumulation is constantly high in the interstitium; the macrophages contain lipid droplets and siderosomes (OLSZEWSKI 1977). The connective tissue may be characterized by cracking and a decrease in number of the elastic fibers (SCHNEIDER et al. 1968). The collagen fibers can be detached from the endothelial cells (VIRÁGH et al. 1966).

The fibrosclerosis of the interstitial connective tissue gradually transforms the soft stage of manifest lymphedema into the hard, late stage.

14.2.4 Elephantiasis

The hyperkeratotic verrucous thickening of the epidermis and the fibrosclerotic alteration of the dermis transform the extremities until they become elephantoid.

The most severe elephantoid skin changes are seen in filariasis, but elephantiasis is not synonymous with filariasis. Elephantiasis is the most severe morphological stage of chronic lymphostatic edema. It can have various causes.

The name "elephantiasis nostras" has been used to distinguish these cases from ones of true tropical elephantiasis, which is a filarial disease. It seems practical to use the adjectival form, "elephantoid", to describe the characteristic picture of lymphedema with hyperkeratotic epidermal changes and fibrosis of the dermis.

14.3 Inflammatory Skin Conditions Leading to Chronic Lymphedema

14.3.1 Usual Forms

Recurrent skin infections accompanied by lymphangitis are followed by a progressive lymphedema.

In lymphedema accompanied by the post-thrombophlebitic syndrome and leg ulcers, the leading factor is that the lymphatic load exceeds the lymphatic transport capacity. The high lymph-flow failure is aggravated by chronic infection of the ulcers, recurrent episodes of elephantiasis, and occasional episodes of eczematous lesions.

Following injury the high regenerating capacity of the lymphatic vessel may be disturbed by infection, thrombosis, scar formation, or inflammation (post-traumatic lymphedema) (OLSZEWSKI 1977).

14.3.2 Rare Forms

Elephantoid enlargement of the ears is a rarely described form of lymphedema. It is the consequence of repeated inflammatory events of eczema, pediculosis capitis, frostbite, and erysipelas (MAHZOON and AZADEH 1983).

Chronic vulvitis is the result of recurring furunculosis of the labia majora accompanied by lymphocytic vulvitis. The histological picture resembles that of cheilitis granulomatosa (LARSSON and WESTERMARK 1978).

Severe lymphedema of the hand has been documented after recurrent lymphangitis and infections as unusual complications of allergic contact dermatitis (after a long period) of the hands. Skin infections can lead to increased inflammatory processes in eczema (LYNDE and MITCHELL 1982; WORM et al. 1983).

14.4 Diagnosis of Lymphostatic Edema

The diagnosis of lymphedema rests on a careful clinical history and physical examination and occasionally on lymphangiography. In lymphangiography with the "naked eye", the specific dye of patent blue violet appears electively in the lymphatic vessels. Under normal conditions the dye appears in a circumscribed region proximal to the point of the injection. In lymphedema the dye appears in a diffuse reticulate pattern.

Radiological lymphangiography, using contrast medium to make the lymphatic vessels visible, is informative to show malformations, tumors, and the block along the lymphatic being studied.

Isotope lymphangiography with isotope-labeled human albumin is used to follow the protein clearance from the tissues (LINDEMAYR et al. 1984). With fluorescence lymphangiography the lymphatic capillaries and collecting vessels are visible after the injection of fluorescent material (BOLLINGER et al. 1981).

Indirect lymphangiography involves the subepidermal injection of a water-soluble contrast medium that produces staining of the lymphatic capillaries and dermal lymphatics. From a practical point of view, indirect lymphangiography is useful in the diagnosis of lymphedema to discover hypoplasia or hyperplasia of the lymphatic capillaries.

These new methods enhance our knowledge of the pathogenesis of lymphedema and are an aid in planning the therapeutic strategy. In lymphedema lymphangiography can produce a safety-valve insufficiency of the lymph flow leading to much more severe edema and necrosis. All of the invasive diagnostic methods should therefore be employed only if there is a *therapeutic consequence of the examination.*

The pathophysiology of the different classes of edema, their classification and their differential diagnosis have been described in detail in the literature (ALLEN 1934; BRUNNER 1972; FÖLDI 1969; HUTH 1983; MORTIMER and RYAN 1986; RUSZNYÁK et al. 1967).

The histological structure and the elctron-microscopical ultrstructure of lymphostatic edema are not yet clearly understood. This is due to a relative neglect of morphological research in this area.

Here we will be concerned with the structural and electron-microscopical details of the dermal lymphatic capillaries in lymphostatic edema in man.

14.5 Histological and Electron-Microscopical Features of Lymphostatic Edema

The proliferation of the lymphatic vessels as a dynamic adaptation to lymphostasis has been described in experimental studies (CLODINS 1977; OLSZEWSKI 1977).

Ectatic lymphatic capillaries are seen in the reticular dermis, beneath the edematous connective tissue of the papillary dermis. The small blood vessels are also dilated (PFLEGER 1964a).

We observed ectatic lymphatic capillaries in the middle dermis of patients suffering from bilateral lymphostatic edema of the lower limb. Besides the clinical and histological symptoms of lymphedema in these cases, lymphangioma circumscriptum-like tumors could be demonstrated as long-term complications of chronic lymphedema.

A 57-year-old female patient (case 1) was operated on for uterine cancer and irradiated with roentgen rays. After 6 years she developed bilateral irreversible lymphedema of her lower limbs. The non-pitting lymphedema was complicated by temporary lymphorrhea after minor traumas, superficial necrotic plaques, and circumscribed lymphangioma-like tumors (Figs. 116 and 117). Recurring episodes of erysipelas were also mentioned in the anamnesis. One of the biopsied tumors proved histologically to be acquired lymphangiectasis.

Case 2 illustrates isolated elephantoid changes of the toe. A 61-year-old female patient had suffered a left shin-bone fracture. Three years after this injury she began to complain of burning pains and temporary pitting edema of the left leg. Six years after the bone fracture we admitted her to the clinic to treat the unilateral lower limb non-pitting chronic lymphedema and the isolated elephantoid changes of the second toe. The skin of the swollen indurated toe was hyperkeratotic and the fibrotic hyperplasia gave it a cauliflower-like appearance (Fig. 118). The histological examination showed the morphological characteristics of acquired lymphangiectasis (Fig. 119).

In acquired lymphangiectasis also called "acquired lymphangioma", the epidermal surface is hyperkeratotic. The long epidermal ridges protrude deeply into the compact papillary dermis. The collagen bundles are increased in number; they seem to be homogeneous. The elastic fibers are diminished. The blood capillaries are also increased in number and their endothelial wall is thick. Mononuclear cells are revealed in the upper dermis. The skin appendages are missing. In the middle and deep dermis dilated lymphatic vessels are present. A short stem of the valves protrudes into the lymphatic lakes, the endothelial cells are not increased or hypertrophic, and the lymphatic wall is surrounded by connective tissue. The wall does not possess smooth muscle cells; the vessels represent lymphatic capillaries (Fig. 119).

Under the electron microscope the dermal lymphatic capillaries are seen to be dilated. The attenuated endothelial cells are connected with each other by overlapping (Figs. 120 and 121) and end-to-end junctions (Fig. 126). Gaps or open junctions between the endothelial cells have also been observed. The organelle content of the endothelial cells proved to be different along the capillary wall. The elongated narrow processes are poorly contrasted; they contain some pinocytotic vesicles and polyribosomes (Figs. 120–122, 126 and 127).

The perinuclear cytoplasm is rich in organelles: mitochondria, modest amounts of endoplasmic reticulum, and Golgi complexes can be observed. The nuclei are oval or indented.

The numbers of the pinocytotic and intracytoplasmic vesicles are decreased in comparison with normal conditions or with acute inflammation (Figs. 123, 124, 128).

Tubular microfilaments measuring 10–12 nm in diameter and anchoring the abluminal membrane of the endothelial cells to the connective tissue have not been found. This observation contrasts with that of ALTORFER and CLODINS (1976), who reported an increased number of connective-tissue mcirofilaments around the lymphatic capillaries of dogs in chronic experimental lymphedema. They frequently found fibrin thrombi in the lymphatic vessels in the latent and chronic phases of lymphedema. In our patients with chronic lymphedema, fibrin thrombi have been rarely encountered in the lymphatic capillary lumen.

The basal lamina material is increased along the short segments of the lymphatic capillaries (Figs. 124, 132, 137), but in general a continuous basal lamina is lacking.

The lymphatic capillaries are surrounded by granulofilamentous material. The cotton-like substance resembling the content of the capillary lumen envelops the connective tissue fibers (Figs. 120–122).

A direct contact between the lymphatic capillary endothelium and the connective tissue fibers does not exist. The collagen and elastic fibers are located apart from the lymphatic endothelium. The granulofilamentous material occupies the periendothelial space (Figs. 120–122, 128, 136). The perivascular space is occupied by fibroblasts (Fig. 127) and connective tissue cells with the ultrastructural features of both fibroblasts and myoblasts. They are called "myofibroblasts". They are surrounded by basal lamina material. Pinocytotic vesicles are revealed along the cell membrane, and the cytoplasm contains numerous mitochondria and prominent tubules of endoplasmic reticulum. Compact bundles of actomyosin filaments displaying regular densities are demonstrated along the cell periphery (Figs. 123, 124, 126, 131) and in the cytoplasm (Fig. 125).

The amount of microfilamentous ground substance is increased, and in some places the perivascular space is full of star-shaped glycosaminoglycan-rich fibrils (Fig. 129).

Branching connective-tissue microfilaments measuring about 10 nm in diameter are intermingled with the collagen fibers (Fig. 130), creating a long-spaced periodic pattern (Fig. 131).

The pericapillary elastic fibers demonstrate different forms of elastic degeneration. The elastic microfilaments are diminished in number. The surface of the fragmented elastotic material seems to be "hairy" due to the tiny attaching filaments (Fig. 132). The elastotic dense spots puncturing the granular elastotic substance give a leopard-like appearance to the pathological elastic fiber (Fig. 133). The third variant of the degeneration elastica, consisting

of dense fuzzy granules, looks like a string of pearls (Figs. 134 and 135). The collagen fibers vary in diameter from 10 to 200 nm. Some of the thin and thick variants seem to be twisted around their longitudinal axis. The flower-like cross sections of these variants show the disorganization of the collagen fibers (Fig. 136).

The collagen flower represents a unique structural abnormality of the dermal collagen fibers, which can be observed in various connective-tissue disorders (HOLBROOK and BYERS 1982).

In lymphostatic edema the protein content of the interstitial fluid is high and biochemical composition of the perilymphatic ground substance is changed. The polymerization of the connective tissue fibers is altered, and various structural abnormalities can be discovered (DARÓCZY 1986). We found the characteristic collagen abnormalities (thin and thick fibers, collagen flowers) not only in lymphostatic edema but also in lymphangioma circumscriptum (Fig. 137) and in chronic dermal infiltration (Figs. 138 and 139).

Following is a summary of the ultrastructural features of lymphedema:

1. The epidermis is acanthotic, the ridges are elongated, and the surface is covered by a multilayered stratum corneum.
2. The papillary connective tissue is compact; the collagen bundles are thick and seem to be homogeneous. The elastic fibers are diminished in number.
3. The blood capillaries are increased in number and they have a thick wall.
4. The skin appendages are diminished in number or absent.
5. Mononuclear cells are seen around the vessels and scattered in the papillary dermis. The macrophages are lacking.
6. The lymphatic capillaries are seen in the middle and deep dermis; they are dilated. The short valve structures protrude into the lake-like lymphatic lumen.
7. The thickness of the endothelial cells, the number of types of intercellular junctions, and the organelle content of the cytoplasm vary according to the functional stage of the section studied.

8. The basal lamina is discontinuous, at some places folded several times.
9. Microfilaments 10–20 nm in diameter anchoring the abluminal endothelial surface of the endothelial cells to the connective tissue are lacking.
10. The connective-tissue microfilaments 11–13 nm in diameter are increased in number.
11. The perivascular space is filled with loose granulofilamentous material showing the same electron density as the contents of the lymphatic lumen.
12. Myofibroblasts with the morphological features of both fibroblasts and smooth muscle cells are found around the lymphatic capillaries.
13. The connective tissue ground substance in the perilymphatic area is very rich in glycosaminoglycans, showing star-like microfilaments.
14. The elastic fibers show varying forms of degeneration. There are fewer elastic microfilaments.
15. Long-spacing collagen, thin and thick fibers (10–200 nm in diameter), and twisted or flower-like variants represent the different structural abnormalities of the collagen fibers.

Fig. 116. Lymphedema, case 1. Superficial necrotic plaques are seen over the shin *(star)*. Hyperkeratotic skin covers the fibrotic swollen masses around the ankle *(arrow)* divided by deep wrinkles

Fig. 117. Close-up of the shin (case 1). Numerous lymphangioma-like yellowish or skin-colored soft tumors *(arrows)* are seen on the lower leg

Fig. 118. Lymphedema, case 2. The second elephantoid toe of the left foot is congested. The papillomatous surface is hyperkeratotic

Fig. 119. Acquired lymphatic hyperplasia or reactive lymphangiectasis (case 2). Beneath the acanthotic epidermis the papillary collagen bundles are compact; the elastic fibers are missing. In the middle dermis the lymphatic lakes are formed by dilated lymphatic capillaries. H and E, × 100

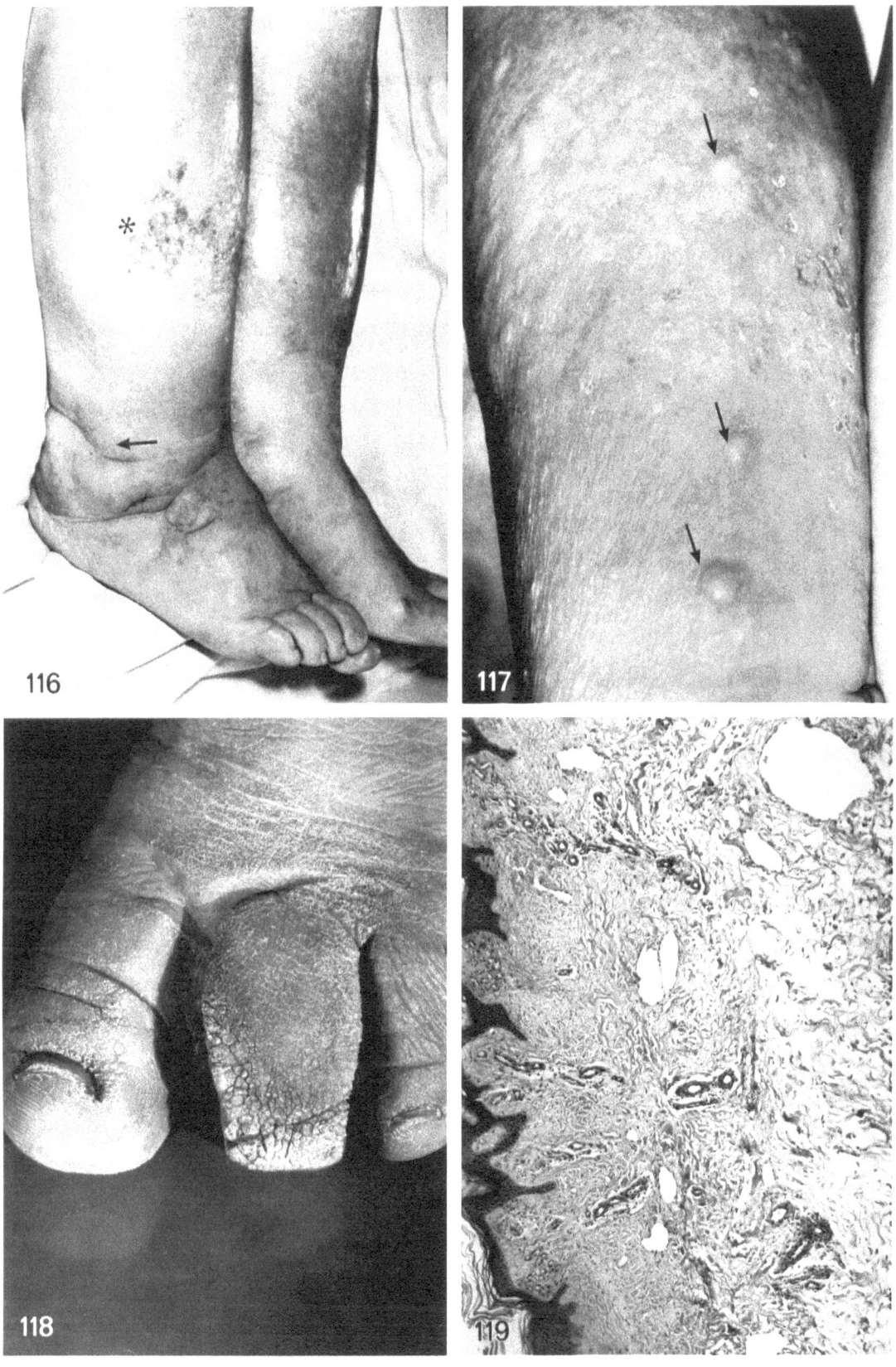

Fig. 120. Lymphedema, human lower leg. Endothelial processes range into the dilated lumen *(Lu)*. The intercellular junction – inlet valve – seems to be open *(arrow)*. Between the endothelial wall and the collagen coat around the lymphatic capillary, the subendothelial space *(star)* is filled with a fine granulofilamentous substance of plasma density. *F,* Fibroblast; × 4000

Fig. 121. Lymphedema, human lower leg. The lympahtic endothelial cell *(End)* contains numerous pinocytotic vesicles. The loose structure of the perilymphatic space consists of fine granulofilamentous material intermingled with some collagen fibers and remnants of elastic fibers *(E)*. The collagen bundles around the lymphatic capillary display numerous flower-like individual fibers *(arrow)*. × 7000

Fig. 122. Lymphedema, human lower limb. The wide perilymphatic space *(star)* filled with granulofilamentous material showing the same electron density as the lymph in the lumen *(Lu)* separates the endothelial wall *(End)* from the collagen *(Co)* bed around the lymphatic capillary. × 4800

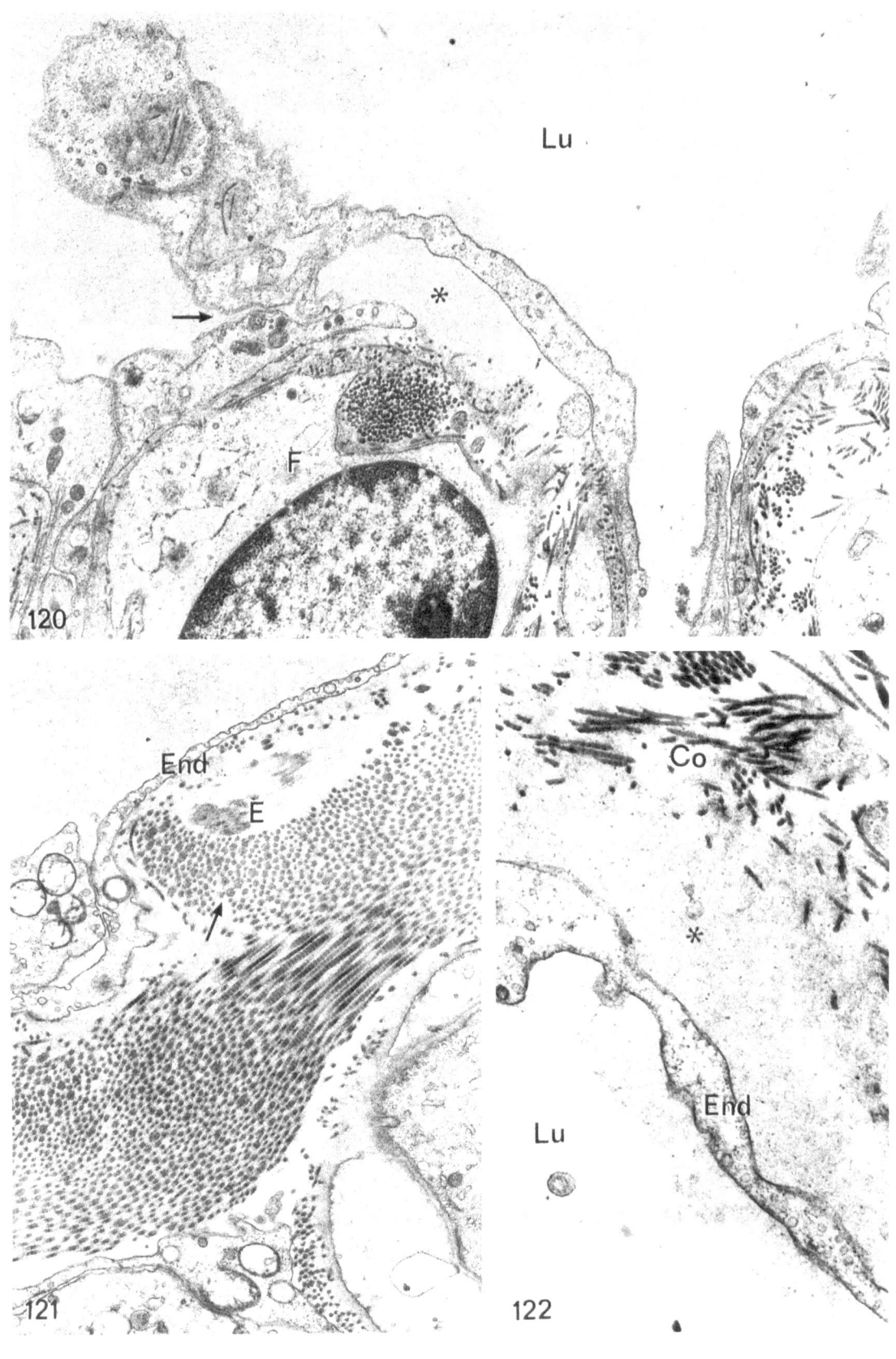

Fig. 123. Lymphedema, human lower leg. The cytoplasm of the endothelial cell *(End)* is rich in organelles. The perilymphatic space of the capillary *(stars)* contains granulofilamentous material and some collagen fibers. In the perilymphatic interstitium there are fibroblasts *(F)* with dense filamentous plates along the cytoplasmic membranes *(arrows).* × 4800

Fig. 124. Lymphedema, human lower leg. The basal lamina-like material is multiplied *(Bl)* around the lymphatic capillary. The cytoplasmic process of the perivascular fibroblast *(F)*, containing numerous mitochondria *(Mi)*, is characterized by the dense bundle of filaments *(arrow)* running along the cell membrane. × 7200

Fig. 125. Lymphedema, human lower leg. Detail of a myofibroblast possessing well-developed endoplasmic cisternae *(Er)* and filamentous bundle with periodic densities *(arrows).* The perilymphatic cell infiltrate is composed of neutrophilic leukocytes *(Leu)* and macrophages *(Ma).* × 2500

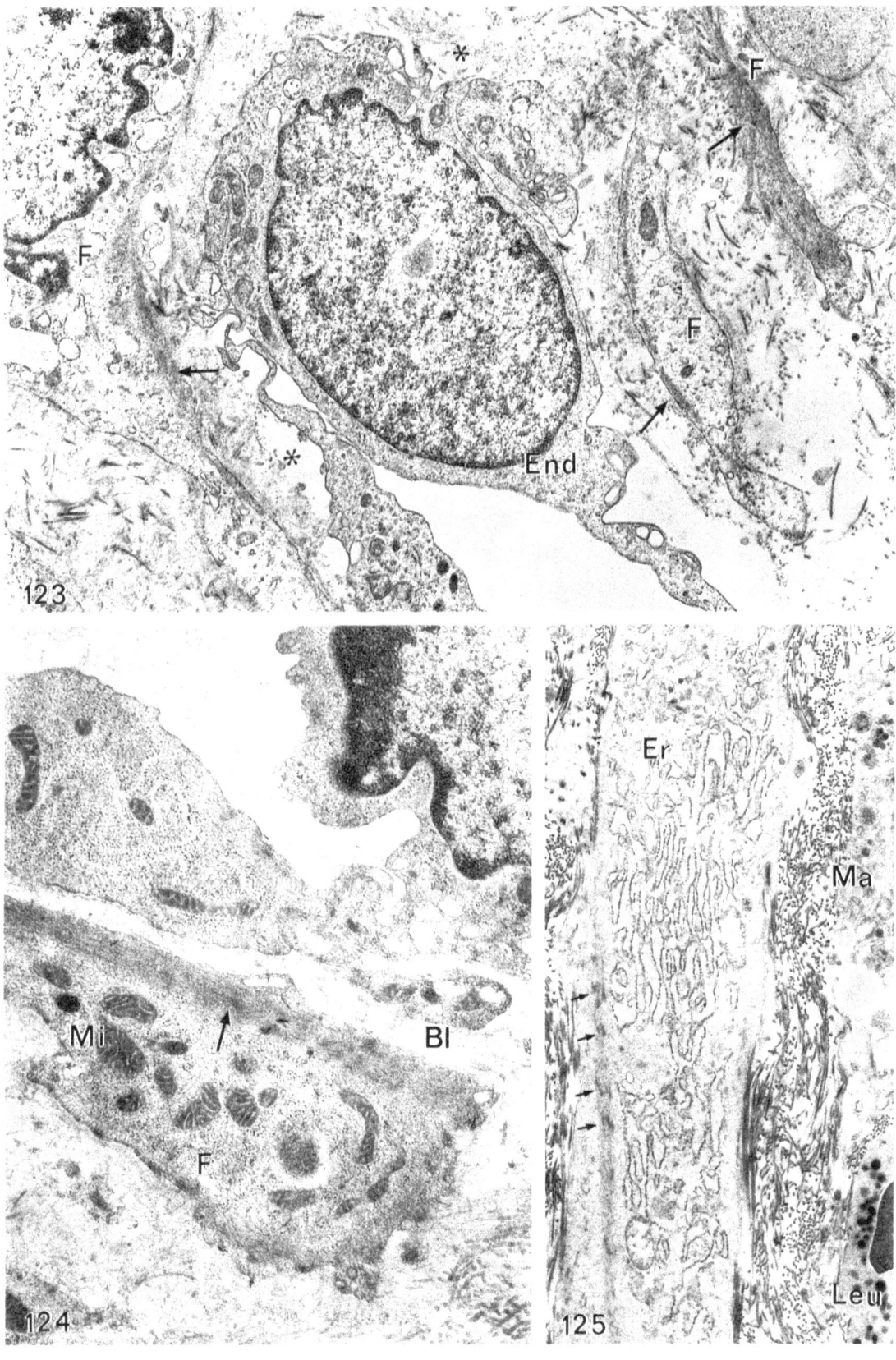

Fig. 126. Lymphedema, human lower leg. An end-to-end intercellular junction *(arrow)* connects the endothelial cell processes to each other. The cytoplasmic detail of the perilymphatic myofibroblast possesses a dense peripheral bundle *(star)* of fine filaments. *Lu,* Lymphatic lumen; × 12500

Fig. 127. Lymphedema, human lower leg. The overlapping *(arrow)* flat endothelial processes of the lymphatic capillary are connected directly with the perilymphatic space. The fibroblast *(F)* is in close vicinity to the capillary wall. × 4800

Fig. 128. Lymphedema, human lower leg. The endothelial cells surrounding the dilated lymphatic lumen *(Lu)* are thin at some sections of the wall, but at the adjacent portion the cytoplasm buds into the lumen and contains prominent organelles, Golgi apparatus *(Go),* and centrioles *(Ce).* The perilymphatic space consists of loose connective-tissue ground substance and collagen fibers. × 5500

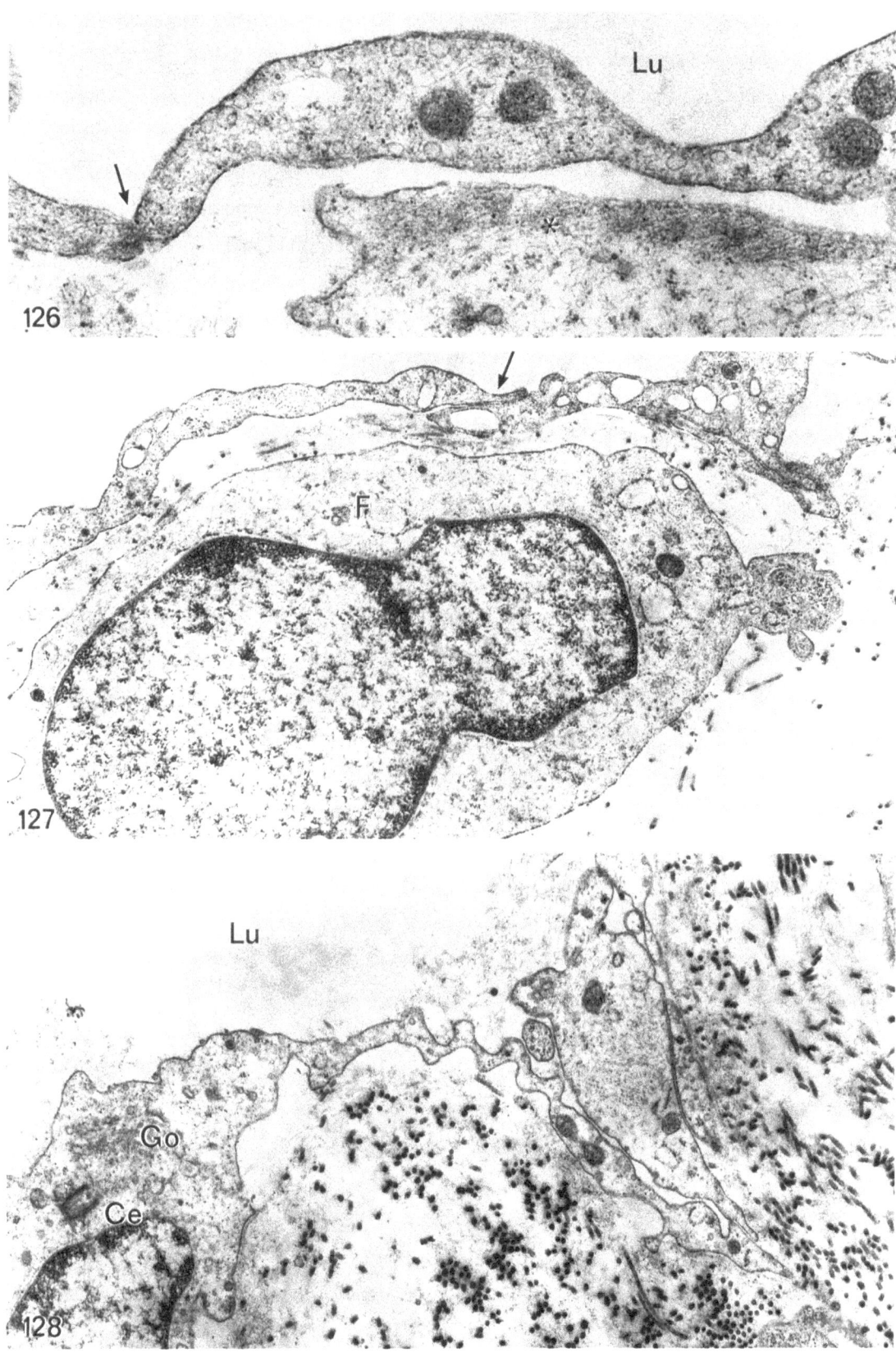

Fig. 129. Lymphedema, human lower leg. The granulofilamentous perivascular space seems to be foamy due to the starlike fibrillar variations of the ground substance. × 10000

Fig. 130. Lymphedema, human lower leg. The flat endothelial cell process is connected with the fragment of basal lamina *(Bl)* or in direct contact with the connective tissue filaments *(f)* measuring 11–12 nm in diameter. The filaments are intermingled with collagen fibers. × 20000

Fig. 131. Lymphedema, human lower leg. The connective tissue around the lymphatic capillary *(L)* is characterized by loose ground substance and long-spacing collagen *(LSC)* variants. The perivascular space is occupied by myofibroblasts with a dense filamentous cytoplasmic bundle *(arrow)*. × 6400

Fig. 132. Lymphedema, human lower leg. The attenuated endothelial cells showing accordion-like undulations are directly connnected with granulofilamentous ground substance surrounded by dense fragments of degenerated perivascular elastic fibers *(E)*. × 10600

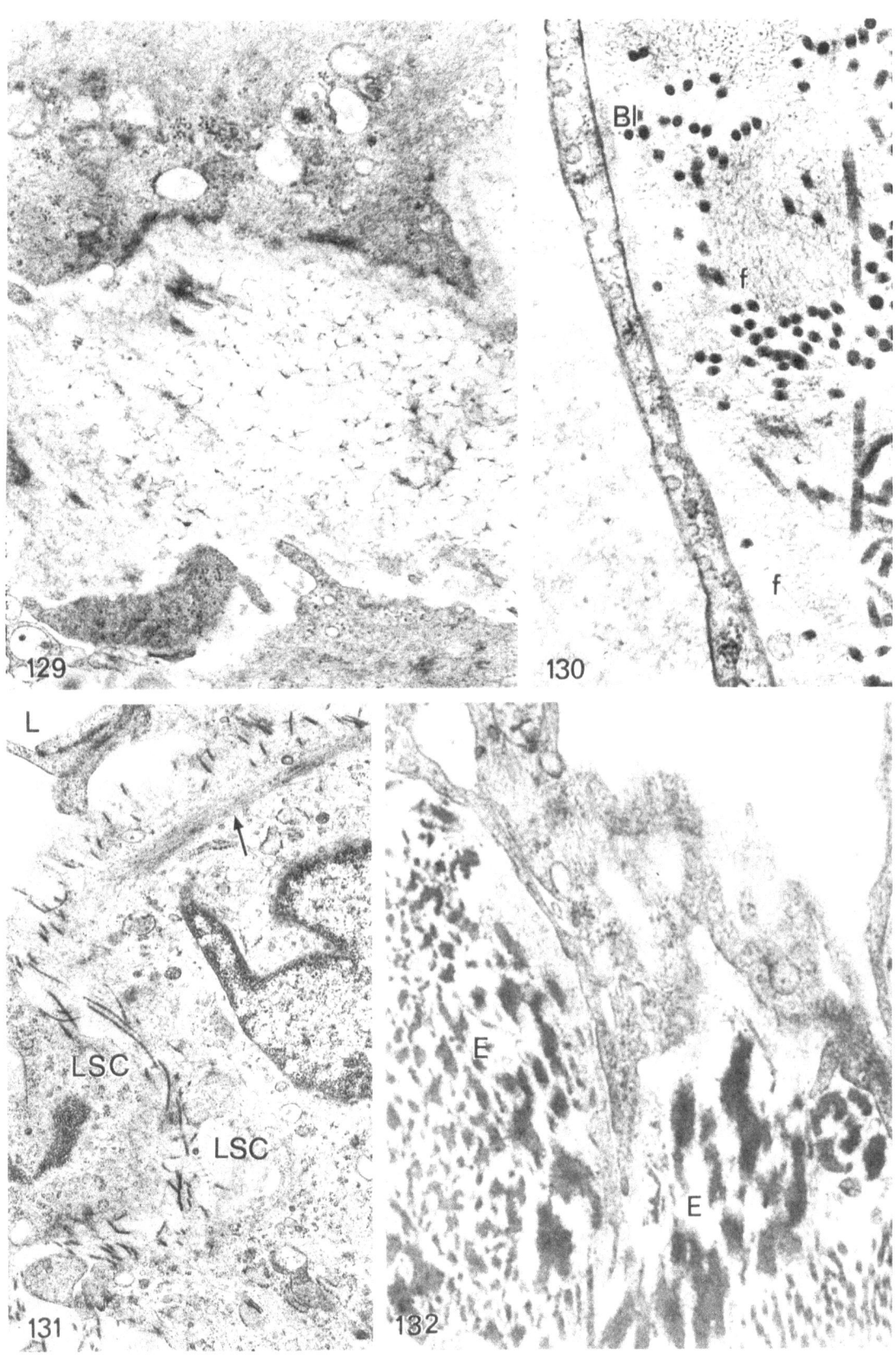

Fig. 133. Lymphedema, human lower leg. The elastic microfilaments are missing around the cross and longitudinal sections of the degenerated perilymphatic elastic fibers. The elastotic material is finely granulated. × 9000

Fig. 134. Lymphedema, human lower leg. The fragmented elastic fibers between the pericapillary fibroblasts *(F)* are intermingled with the granulofilamentous ground substance. × 10000

Fig. 135. Lymphedema, human lower leg. Close-up of the degenerated and fragmented elastic fibers from the perivascular connective tissue. The disintegrated components of the elastic fibers are arranged like strings of pearls. × 33000

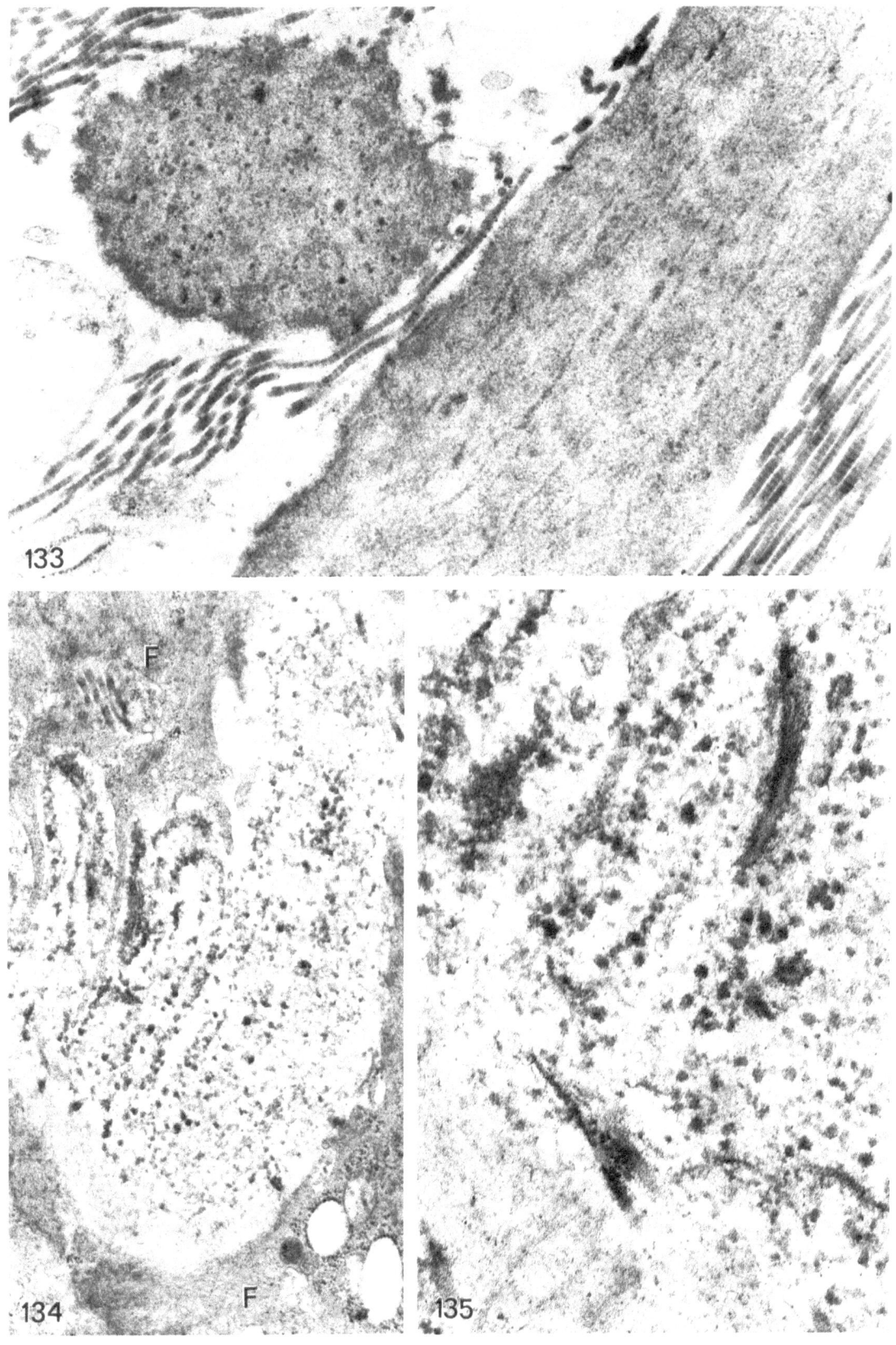

Fig. 136. Lymphedema, human lower leg. The dilated lymphatic capillary *(L)* is separated from the perivascular collagen bundles by a narrow electron-lucent area containing micro-filaments and fragments of elastic fibers *(E)*. The thick, twisting collagen fibers have flower-like cross sections *(arrows)*. × 10 000

Fig. 137. Lymphangioma circumscriptum, human skin, chest wall. The lymphatic endothelial cells are accompanied by interrupted fragments of the basal lamina *(Bl)*. In the perilymphatic region extremely thick collagen bundles are mixed with thin collagen variants and elastic fibers *(E)*. *Lu,* Lymphatic lumen; × 7200

Fig. 138. Lymphangioma circumscriptum, human lower leg. Cross sections of a group of perilymphatic collagen fibers demonstrate the different diameters (30–150 nm) and the flower-like surface of the thick fibers. × 10 600

Fig. 139. Lymphedema, hyperkeratosis, human lower leg. Thin 10 nm and thick 150 nm *(arrow)* variants of collagen fibers are seen around the dermal lymphatic capillary *(L)*. × 3200

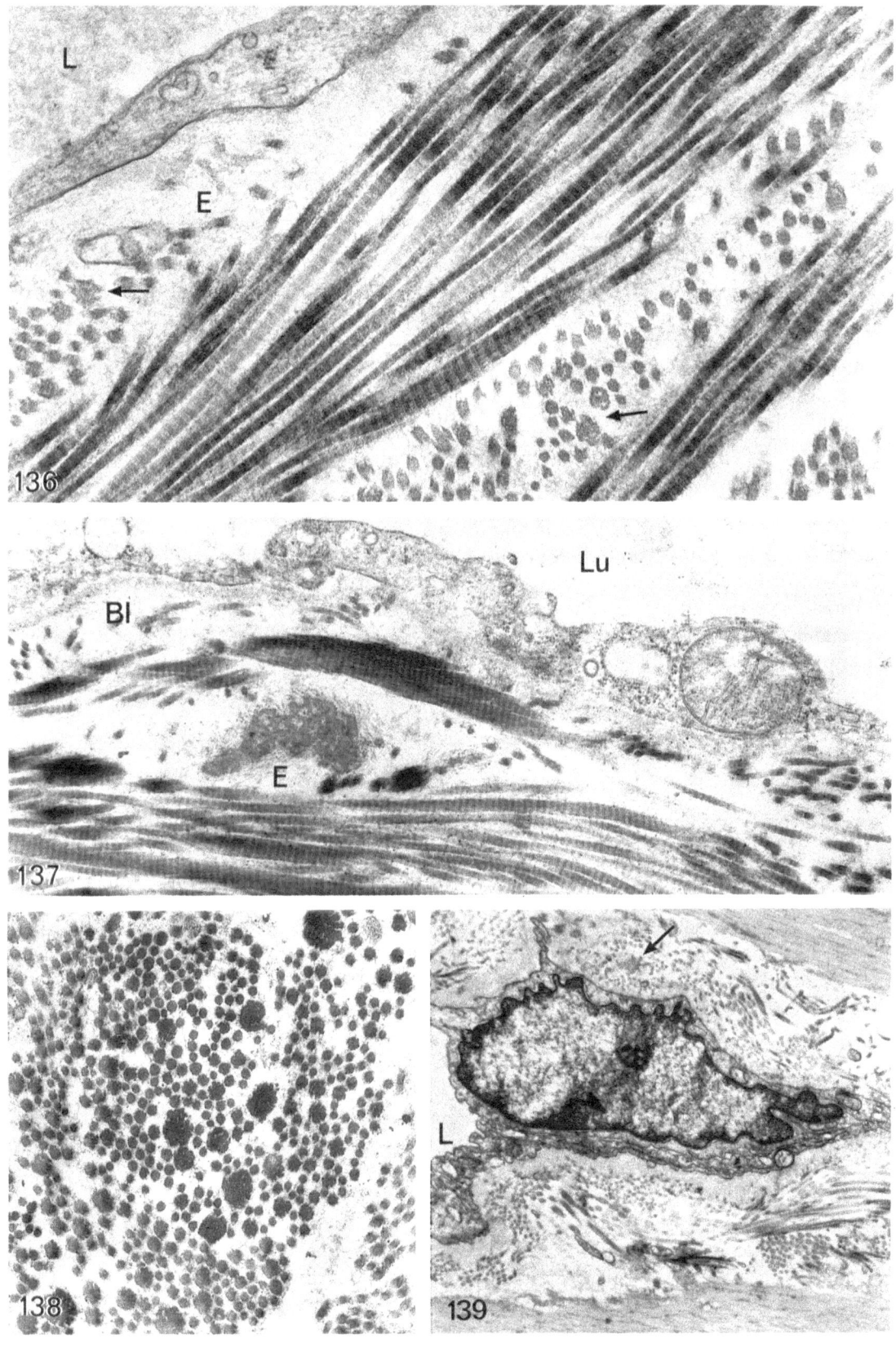

15 Tumors of the Dermal Lymphatics

15.1 Lymphangioma

Lymphangioma circumscriptum is an uncommon, benign, hamartomatous malformation involving primarily the dermal lymphatics and occasionally the subcutaneous vessels.

The lymphangioma may become infiltrative but usually does not undergo malignant transformation (PEACHEY et al. 1970; POSTACCHINI and SADUN 1976). The main regions involved are the internal chest area, the neck, the axilla, the oral cavity, the groin, and the mediastinum. The lymphangioma may appear at any age.

Lymphangioma circumscriptum appears clinically as multiple, small vesicle-like white-to-purple lesions or as small wartlike lesions scattered over a circumscribed skin area. The superficial dilated lymphatics can be connected and partly disconnected, with large lymphatic cisternae lying deep in the subcutis (WHIMSTER 1976), and sometimes they are associated with diffuse swelling in the adjacent subcutis.

Lymphangiomata may originate (a) from sequestration of primitive lymphatic anlagen, (b) as a consequence of congenital absence or blockage of the lymphatic vessels, or (c) due to the incompetence of lymphatic vessels or lymphatic valves (ASANO et al. 1978). The majority of lymphangiomata are congenital in origin.

15.1.1 Congenital

The growth of the tumor and the progressive accumulation of fluid are due to insufficient drainage of lymph from the dilated channels. The tumor is composed of enlarged, dilated lymphatic vessels located immediately beneath the epidermis. The anastomosing cavernous channels of varying size mostly contain a pink-staining material. The walls of the channels are lined by a single layer of endothelial cells (FLANAGAN and HELWIG 1977; PALMER et al. 1978). The complicated vascular labyrinth of the lymphangioma appears on the section plane as a polyploid papillary structure floating in cystic spaces that are lined by proliferating endothelial cells. This peculiar endothelial proliferation can imitate angiosarcoma but the cell anaplasia, necroses, and mitoses of that condition are missing (KUO and GOMEZ 1979). Erythrocytes and lymphocytes are usually seen in the lumen of the proliferating lymphatics.

To avoid confusion in the classification of lymphangiomata, (FLANAGAN and HELWIG (1977) use only two basic types in their practical diagnosis: (a) lymphangioma circumscriptum and (b) deep lymphangioma cavernosum. In the latter condition, hygromata arise from the jugular lymph sacs and are found mainly in the region of the neck, axilla, or breast, and they are associated with diffuse swelling of the adjacent subcutaneous tissue. Hemangioma and lymphangioma are frequently combined.

Lymphangiomata may be treated successfully by excising the subcutaneous cisternae without removing the overlying skin. However, the tumors can reappear repeatedly.

In a present case (case 3) of lymphangioma circumscriptum the 23-year-old female patient had some yellowish tumors in the right scapular region since birth. In her late teens the color of the tumors became reddish and numerous new tumors have since developed over her chest wall (Fig. 140).

The main histological characteristic, as reported elsewhere in the literature, (FLANAGAN and HELWIG 1977, PEACHEY et al. 1970) was the dilated channels of the anastomosing lymphatics situated immediately beneath the epidermis. Erythrocytes occurred in the lumen and orcein-positive elastic fibers were observed in the vessel wall (Fig. 141).

Under the electron microscope the endothelial cells of the lymphatic capillary were seen protruding into the lumen; their nuclei were indented and the cytoplasm contained bundles of filaments and well-developed endoplasmic reticulum.

Tubuloreticular structures consisting of reticular aggregates of membranous tubules were not infrequent inclusions located within the cisternae of endoplasmic reticulum (Figs. 142 and 143). The lymphatic capillary was accompanied by multilayered basal lamina and basal lamina-like material. The collagen fibers, varying in diameter, showed numerous flower-like forms on cross sections. The microfilamentous component of the elastic fibers was very prominent (Figs. 142 and 144).

15.1.2 Acquired

Acquired lymphatic dilatations appear secondarily, provokated by an identifiable cause. Trauma can favor the development of lymphangioma by causing blockage in the lymphatic drainage system.

Lymphangioma seems to be induced by lymphostasis in some cases and is considered a complication of long standing lymphedema (cf. case 1).

The acquired forms of lymphangioma may result from lymphatic obstruction due to irradiation, trauma, tumor, infection, or recurrent infections of erysipelas, filariasis, or tuberculosis. HEUVEL et al. (1979) described lymphangiectasis of the vulva appearing as clear vesicles on the labia majora in a patient with lymph node tuberculosis of both groins. The patient also had a swollen left leg. Repeated episodes of tuberculous lymphadenitis of the axilla (DiLEONARDO and JACOBY 1986) were followed by lymphangiomata on the chest wall.

Lymphangiomata have been reported in association with tumor metastasis to the regional lymph nodes (WEAKLEY and JUHLIN 1961) and on the vulva of a female patient several years

after irradiation for squamous carcinoma of the cervix uteri (FISCHER and ORKIN 1970).

Histologically, dilated lymphatics are present beneath the epidermis and in the mid dermis in acquired lymphangioma. The lymph vessels contain lymphocytes and erythrocytes imparting a reddish tingle or deep purple color to the lesions. Surgical removal of the lymphatic tumors is adequate treatment.

15.2 Lymphangiosarcoma (Stewart-Treves Syndrome)

STEWART and TREVES (1948) reported the first six cases of lymphangiosarcoma arising from long-standing secondary surgical lymphedema that had followed radical mastectomy. They termed the tumor "postmastectomy lymphangiosarcoma". A review of the literature shows several cases of lymphangiosarcoma arising on congenitally or postoperatively lymphedematous extremities (LASKAS et al. 1975). Continuous monitoring of patients with primary and secondary lymphedema is necessary because of the high risk of lymphangiosarcoma.

Following the report by STEWART and TREVES it was accepted that the tumor derived from lymphatic endothelial cells. Other authors have described it as a tumor of blood vessels or as a mixed vascular tumor with lymphatic participation.

In the tumor the anastomosing and labyrinth-like channels are lined by swollen hyperchromatic endothelial cells budding into the lumen. The endothelial cells can form intraluminal tufts. The occurrence of factor VIII-related antigen in the tumor cells indicates that the tumor is more likely a hemangiosarcoma than a lymphangiosarcoma (SCHMITZ-RIXEN et al. 1984).

Ultrastructurally, the tumorous endothelial cells and pericytes show strong similarities with Kaposi's sarcoma. The tumor cells contain well-developed endoplasmic reticulum, Golgi complexes, free ribosomes, and large amounts of glycogen particles (SILVERBERG et al. 1971). There are documented cases in which hemangiosarcoma was indistinguishable from postmastectomy lymphangiosarcoma under the light microscope (REED et al. 1966).

Lymphangiosarcoma arising from lymphangioma circumscriptum has been reported, but in these cases the pre-existing lymphangioma had been exposed to radiation therapy (GIRARD et al. 1970, KING et al. 1979). Rapid regional intervention provides the best prognosis for survival. Early ablative therapy is recommended.

15.3 Pseudo Kaposi's Sarcoma

It can be difficult to differenciate between circumscribed vascular hyperplasia and the early stage of Kaposi's sarcoma. The circumscribed proliferation of the blood vessels is the main morphological change. The dermal lymphatic capillaries play a secondary role in the development of the disease. Clinically, the patients have reddish-brown papules and tumors over a circumscribed area of the extremities that simulate Kaposi's sarcoma. Arteriovenous anastomoses and other vascular malformations can be documented.

The case of a 37-year-old male patient presented here (case 4) began with recurrent episodes of erysipelas affecting the right lower leg. After 2 years a circumscribed angiomatous hyperplasia became manifest over his right shin.

The circumscribed solid plaque seemed to be composed of small light brown papules (Fig. 145). The environment was edematous. Angiography showed no arteriovenous malformations, but the peripheral arteries were tortuous at the site of the skin lesions. Histologically, the epidermis was acanthotic and the vascularity of the papillary dermis was increased. The wall of the blood vessels was thickened and the vascular basal lamina was multiply folded.

Under the electron microscope the swollen endothelial cells of the small arterioles imitated the occlusion of the lumen; the pericytic ring was prominent. Dilated lymphatic capillaries were observed in the mid dermis. The compact collagen bundles of the dermis consisted of thin and thick, 10–150 nm fiber variants. The num-

ber of elastic fibers was diminished in the deeper dermis (Figs. 146 and 147). The fibroblasts seemed to be active, showing prominent tubules and cisternae of endoplasmic reticulum. Extravasated erythrocytes were found frequently. Macrophages loaded with dense lysosomes and some lymphocytes could be observed in the expanded interfibrillary spaces (Fig. 148). The histological changes in pseudo Kaposi's sarcoma closely resemble those of Kaposi's sarcoma: the proliferation of small blood vessels and fibrobalsts, the extravasation of erythrocytes, and the deposition of hemosiderin in the dermis follow the same morphological pattern; however, the characteristic vascular slit pattern seen in Kaposi's sarcoma is absent.

MALI et al. (1965) proposed the term "acroangiodermatitis" for patients with chronic venous insufficiency. RAJKA and KOROSSY (1954) described the disease under the name "neuroangiosis cutis hemosiderica" and suggested that lymphatic hypertrophy might be associated with the angioproliferation. EARHART et al. (1974) use the term "pseudo Kaposi' sarcoma" to call attention to the close similarity of this lesion to Kaposi's sarcoma. Patients about 30 years of age with pseudo Kaposi' sarcoma be examined for an underlying arteriovenous malformation.

15.4 Kaposi's Sarcoma

The primary change in Kaposi's sarcoma is the multifocal neoplastic proliferation of endothelial cells of either blood or lymphatic origin.

The tumors of Kaposi's sarcoma consist of irregular dilated vascular channels and solid areas of spindle cells. The channels separate collagen fibers giving a "dissection of collagen" appearance. The endothelial cells covering the dilated vascular channels are large. They can show evidence of mitosis and they protrude into the lumen. It is sometimes impossible to distinguish abnormal endothelial cells from the normal endothelium without using endothelial markers.

The application of different methods has

helped to clarify the cell origin of this tumor. This progress was enhanced by an increased interest in Kaposi's sarcoma due to its association with the acquired immunodeficiency syndrome (AIDS).

Using endothelial cell markers, factor VIII-related antigen (FVIIIRA) human leukocyte antigen (HLA A, B, C, HLA-DR), lectin-binding antibodies, and monoclonal antibodies (EN 4 and OAL E) which are endothelial-cell specific, investigators have demonstrated evidence for a vascular origin of Kaposi's sarcoma. With regard to the nodular lesions of Kaposi's sarcoma, there is less agreement concerning the origin of proliferating vascular cells. Numerous reports have appeared demonstrating conflicting results regarding the origin of Kaposi's sarcoma. There are several possible reasons for these contradictory results. Cryostat sections are difficult to interpret because of the complex structure of the tumor, different fixation and embedding methods, and the problems with identifying dermal lymphatics. Cold fixation in periodate lysine paraformaldehyde can be used in immunohistochemical studies with monoclonal antibodies (HOLDEN et al. 1986).

Another reason may be incomplete information about the stage of Kaposi's sarcoma that was studied and ignorance of the fact that the nodular lesions of Kaposi's sarcoma are composed of a *vascular,* lymphangiomatous *part* and *spindle cells.* RUTGERS et al. 1986 studied three vascular but not lymphatic endothelial cell-associated antigens in Kaposi's tumors. Vascular spaces weakly express E 92 and OKM 5 antigens, while the spindle cells express them strongly. Rutgers et al. found a strong positivity with FVIIIRA that was absent or focally weakly demonstrable in the spindle-cell component of Kaposi's sarcoma. They suppose a vascular origin for the endothelial cell components of the tumor.

JONES et al. (1986) found that the flattened cells lining the dilated vascular spaces of Kaposi's sarcoma show moderate staining with EN 4 antigen, weak lectin binding with UEA-1, and negative staining with PAL-E and monoclonal anti-FVIIIRA. This reaction profile is identical to that seen in lymphatic endothelium and points to a lymphatic derivation of the vascular spaces of the tumor.

BECKSTEAD et al. (1985) used FVIIIRA, HLA-DR antigen, the enzymes 5-nucleotidase, ATP-ase, and alkaline phosphatase, and lectin binding with UEA-1 and favor a lymphatic origin of Kaposi's sarcoma.

RUSSEL-JONES demonstrated with his coworkers (RUSSEL-JONES et al. 1986) that the areas of spindle cell proliferation show focal staining for FVIIIRA, positive lectin binding with UEA-1, positivity with EN 4, and negative staining reaction with PAL E. These patterns confirm the endothelial origin of the spindle cell component of the tumor.

These studies demonstrate the *phenotypic heterogeneity* of Kaposi's sarcoma. The vascular spaces are of lymphatic origin; the solid part of the tumor is composed of spindle cells with phenotypic expression of blood vessel endothelium (BECKSTEAD et al. 1985, DORFMAN 1984, JONES et al. 1986, RUTGERS et al. 1986).

Analyzing the results of the immunohistochemical studies, one has to consider that the absence of endothelial markers in some parts of Kaposi's sarcoma may signify that the synthetic capability of the neoplastic endothelium is decreased or diminished. The ultrastructure of biopsy specimens form young homosexual men with Kaposi's sarcoma has been compared with that of biopsy specimens from elderly heterosexuals with the same disease. The morphology was found to be the same in both conditions.

Ultrastructurally, the vessels in Kaposi's sarcoma bear a close resemblance to the lymphatic vessels (MCNUTT et al. 1983). The vessels lack the outer layer of pericytes, the basal lamina is discontinuous, and numerous gap junctions are observed between the endothelial cell.

Kaposi's sarcoma is characterized clinically by the frequent occurrence of severe lymphedema without varicose veins, which suggests the functional failure of the lymph circulation.

Lymphangioma-like Kaposi's sarcoma is a unique variant of the tumor. The main feature is the widely dilated anastomosing lymph-filled channels lined by endothelial cells that are generally larger and more numerous than those in normal lymphatics. The vessels lack continuous basal lamina; they have numerous gaps between the endothelial cells (GANGE and WILSON-JONES 1979).

The history of our case 5 began 4 years ago. Skin tumors developed on the left lower leg of a 76-year-old female patient who had suffered a bone fracture of the left tibia 10 years earlier. In the left shin region a circumscribed group of translucent reddish tumors was observed several years after the trauma. The soft tumors measured 0.5–1 cm in diameter. Histologically, dilated lymphatic channels lined by hypertrophic endothelial cells were observed. The case was diagnosed as an acquired lymphangioma (DARÓCZY and RÀCZ 1987).

During the past few years of her regular follow-up examination, reddish-brown tumors have developed and disseminated on both lower extremities (Fig. 149). Histological examination showed the tumors to be composed of angiomatous and solid parts consisting of spindle-shaped cells (Fig. 150).

Besides the hypertrophic blood vessels, some of the proliferating vascular spaces were characterized by the electron-microscopic morphological features of lymphatic capillaries. The swollen endothelial cells protruding into the lumen contained numerous mitochondria and showed mitotic figures. The vascular basal lamina was discontinuous and the elastic fibers, connected directly with the abluminal endothelial surface, displayed different forms of elastotic degeneration (Figs. 151–153).

This case of lymphangioma-like Kaposi's sarcoma demonstrates the difficulty of the differential diagnosis between acquired lymphangioma and Kaposi's sarcoma.

Fig. 140. Lymphangioma circumscriptum, case 3. Multiple small skin-colored vesicles *(arrows)* and groups of wartlike purple to reddish-black tumors (1–3 mm in diameter) are seen over the right scapular region

Fig. 141. Case 3: Cavernous, anastomosing vessels and cystic spaces of lymphatic capillaries are located beneath the acanthotic epidermis. The erythrocytes are demonstrated in the lumen *(star)*. The number of elastic fibers is increased around the lymphatic vessels. Orcein, × 200

Fig. 142. Case 3: The endothelial border of cystic lymphatic sites displays prominent endothelial cells budding into the lumen *(Lu)*. The nuclei are indented and hyperchromatic. The perivascular basal lamina *(Bl)* material is thickened. The collagen fibers have different diameters and show flower-like forms *(arrows)* in cross sections. × 5500

Fig. 143. Case 3: Detail of an endothelial cell from a lymphatic cyst. A tubuloreticular inclusion *(TRS)* connected with the dilated endoplasmic vacuole is present, in addition to a prominent endoplasmic reticulum *(Er)*, mitochondria *(Mi)*, microfilaments *(mf)*, and ribosomes. × 15000

Fig. 144. Case 3: The basal lamina *(Bl)* around the cystic lymphatic vessel *(L)* is thick and multilayered. Thin and thick variants and flower-like modifications of collagen fibers are intermingled with the microfilaments of elastic fibers *(E)*. × 12300

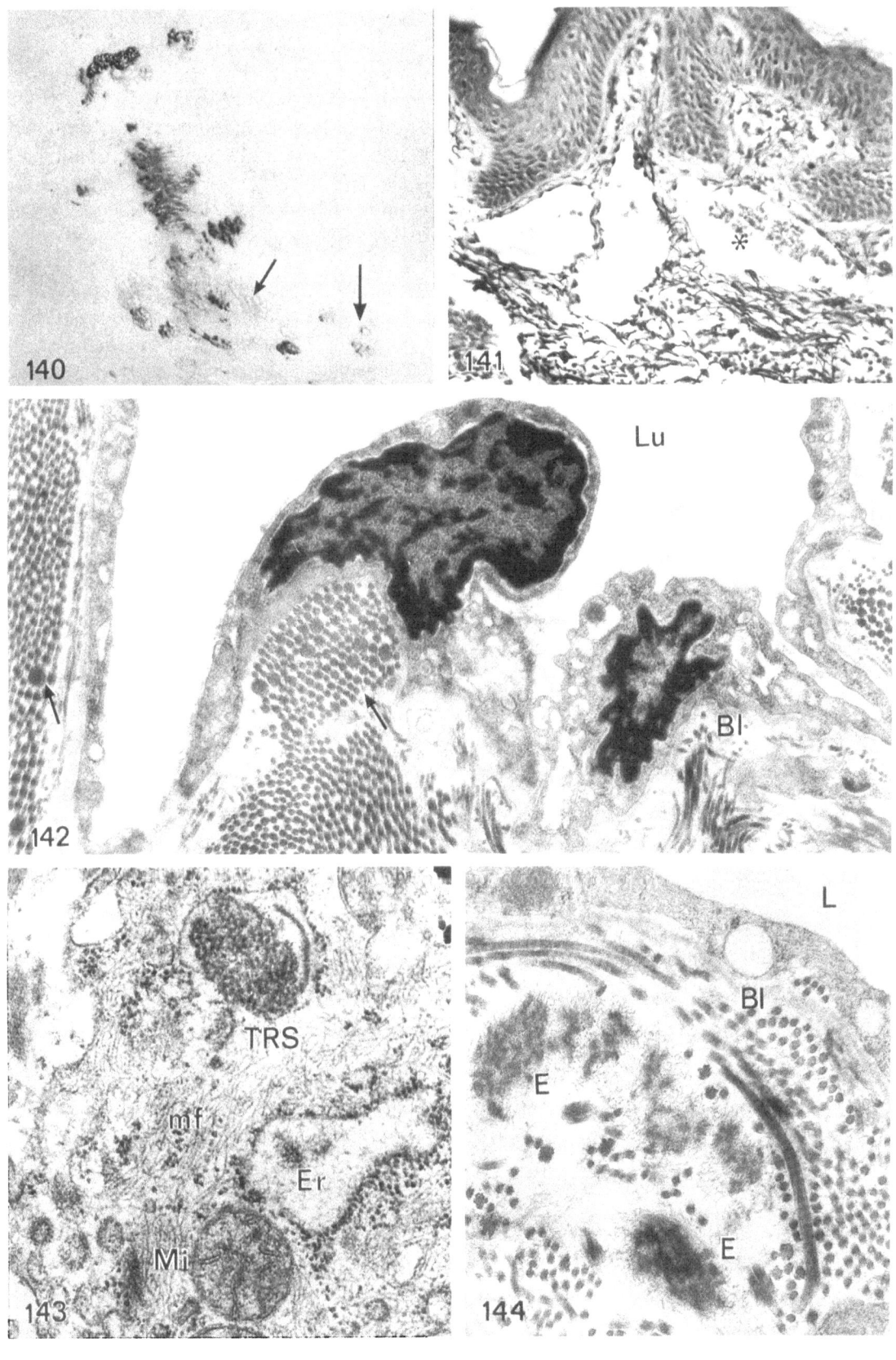

Fig. 145. Pseudo Kaposi's sarcoma, case 4. The left lower leg is edematous. Over the shin there is a brownish, circumscribed plaque composed of small solid papules

Fig. 146. Case 4: The lumen of the dermal arteriole is occluded by the swollen endothelial cells. The multilayered pericytic ring is embedded in the widened basal lamina *(Bl)* material. × 4800

Fig. 147. Case 4: The endothelial cell of the dermal lymphatic capillary is characterized by a long dense plate *(arrow)* composed of fine cytoplasmic filaments 4–5 nm in diameter. The basal lamina is discontinuous. The connective tissue microfilaments *(f)* are increased in number. × 8100

Fig. 148. Case 4: Connective tissue macrophage with phagosomes of different sizes in the cytoplasm. The bizarrely shaped phagosomes are partly membrane bound and show uneven density. × 2500

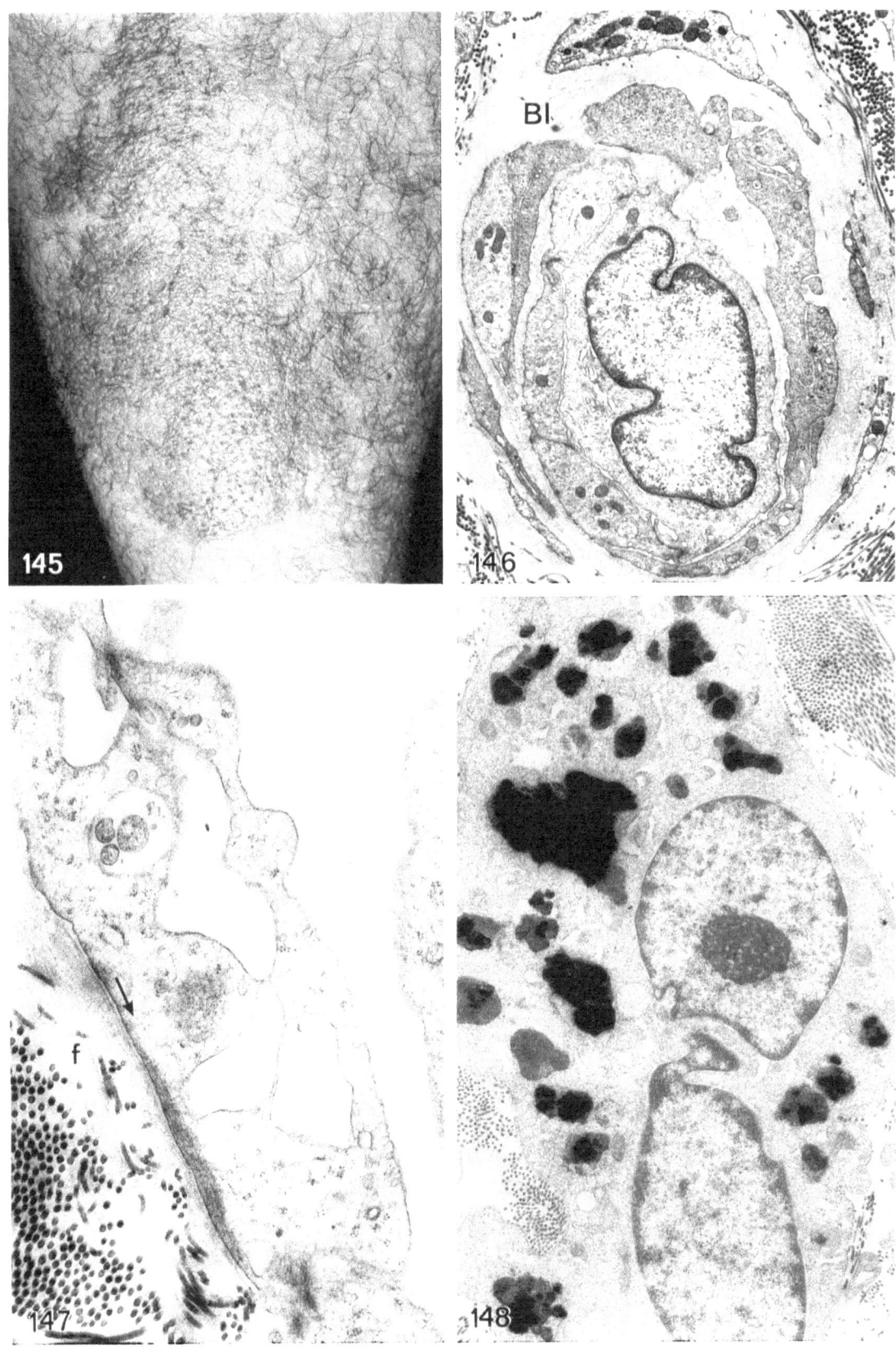

Fig. 149. Kaposi's sarcoma in a 76-year-old female patient, case 5. Reddish-brown tumors are seen on the left lower leg. Some of them show a wrinkled surface and the finger tip sinks into the dermis when the tumors are pressed

Fig. 150. Case 5: The dilated vascular spaces are lined by flat endothelium, but in some places the swollen endothelial cells bud into the lumen *(arrows)*. The vessels are surrounded by nests of spindle-shaped cells. Semithin section; toluidine blue, × 200

Fig. 151. Case 5: A dermal venule *(V)* with swollen endothelial cells, containing numerous dense mitochondria *(Mi)*, is enveloped by multiple folds of basal lamina *(Bl)* and a pericytic layer. The surrounding lymphatic lumen *(Lu)* is lined by thin endothelial cells connected by overlapping *(star)* and end-to-end connections *(arrowhead)*. A continuous basal lamina and the pericytes are missing. × 4800

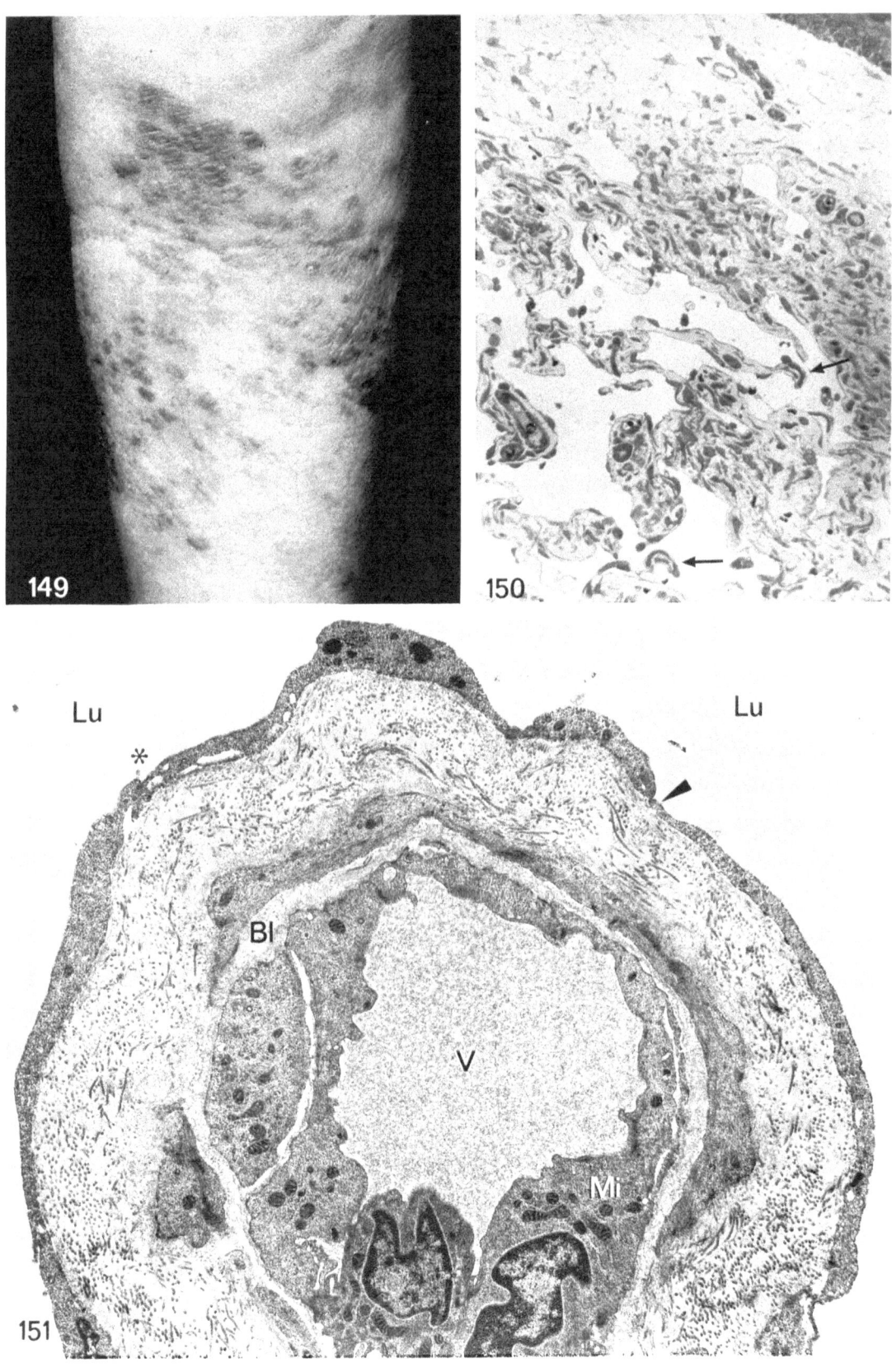

149

150

Lu   Lu

Bl

V

Mi

151

Fig. 152. Kaposi's sarcoma, case 5. A lymphatic endothelial cell containing numerous mitochondria *(Mi)*, dense granules *(g)*, and ribosomes protrudes into the lumen *(Lu)*. The perivascular elastic fibers *(E)* display different forms of elastotic degeneration. The collagen fibers vary in diameter. × 2500

Fig. 153. Case 5: The connective tissue, containing degenerated elastic fibers *(E)* and collagen *(Co)* fibers varying in diameter, is engulfed by one of two endothelial cells *(End$_{1, 2}$)* protruding into the lumen. × 5000

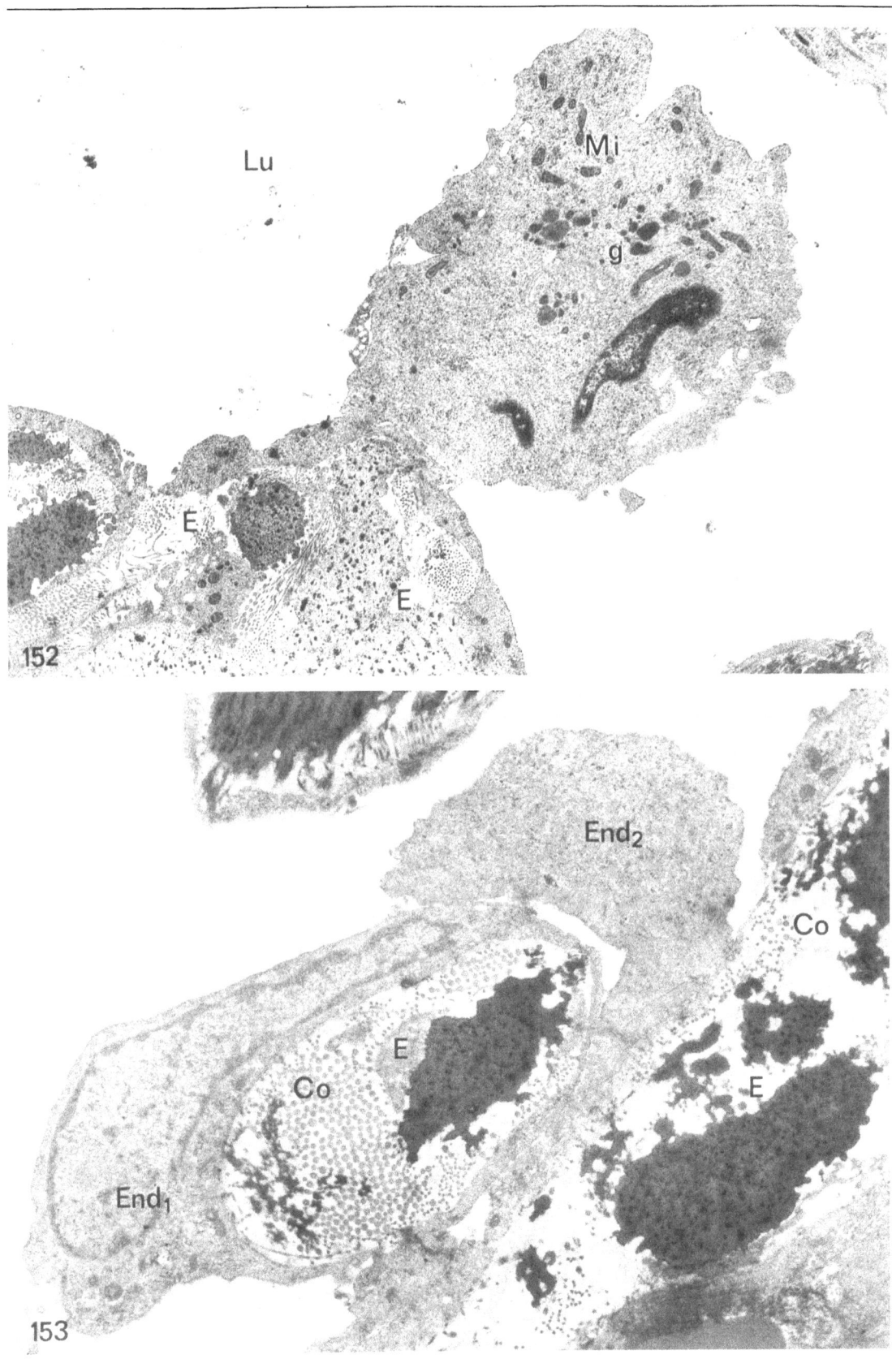

16 Lymphovascular Alterations in Different Syndromes Related to Dermatology

There are clinical syndromes in which lympho-vascular alterations dominate the general syndromatology.

16.1 Melkersson-Rosenthal-Mischer Syndrome

The main features of the triad – edema, facial paresis, and lingua plicata – do not always appear together (MELKERSSON 1928, MISCHER 1945; STORRS 1975). Men and women are affected equally. The first attacks of edema occur in the second to the third decade of life. Low-protein edema is present regularly, with a mild lymphovascular hyperplasia and tuberculoid granulomatous infiltrate. Fibrotic alterations are not essential.

16.2 Klippel-Trenaunay-Weber Syndrome

In this syndrome with vascular dysplasia, nevi flammei, and varices the lymph vessels can participate with ectasia, producing lymphangiomata. The dermal lymph vessels can be aplastic or hypoplastic, resulting in primary lymphedema in some cases (MAY and NISSL 1970).

16.3 Nonne-Milroy-Meige Syndrome

In this syndrome the hyperkeratotic and fibro-sclerotic skin lesions develop as consequences of severe chronic lymphostatic edema due to dysplasia of the lymphovascular system.

16.4 Noonan's Syndrome

This syndrome of hyperkeratosis with Turner's phenotype is characterized by multiple congenital malformations combined with peripheral hypoplasia of the lymphovascular system, resulting in lymphostatic edema.

16.5 Maffucci's Syndrome

Lymphangiomata and lymphangiosarcomata occur often in addition to diffuse symmetric chondromatoses of the bones and unilateral chondrodysplasia, as well as multiple hemangiomata, vitiligo, and pigmented nevi (BEAN 1955).

16.6 Yellow Nail Syndrome

In the background of the syndrome patients have lymphangiomatous alterations in the affected extremities (SAMMAN and WHITE 1964). The nails become thick with keratinous overproduction and the colour turns into yellow. These symptoms are misleading to suppose an onychomycosis and can be the first signs of a lymphatic obstruction.

17 Diabetes mellitus

In this metabolic disorder the lymphatic vessels take part in the development of clinical and morphological symptoms. The pathogenetic tissue processes of organic change involve not only blood vessels but also the lymphatics. OH-KUMA (1979) described a continuous polysaccharide-rich basal lamina (with periodic acid-methenamine staining) around the dermal lymphatics of diabetic patients and hypothesized that it was important for the connective tissue changes. Under normal conditions the dermal lymphatics failed to show a positive basal lamina region by the periodic acid-silver methenamine method, which detects the polysaccharide content.

18 Age-Related Changes of Dermal Lymphatics

Systematic studies of age-related (above the 7th decade) lymphangiosclerosis were carried out on the thoracic duct and large lymphatics. A reduction in tunica media musculature and an increase in collagenous connective tissue were detected.

The fibrotic changes of the large lymphatics did not relate to the degree of general arteriosclerosis.

Age-related reduction of the lymphatic branches was found in the dermis, and a thinner wall and saclike dilatations were observed. The sacculation of the walls was termed "senile varicosity of the lymph vessels" (ZERBINO 1960).

19 Lymphovascular Alterations in Selected Dermatological Diseases

19.1 Porphyria Cutanea Tarda

In the metabolic disease of hemsynthesis pathological changes of the connective tissue are seen. Sclerodermoid clincial symptoms and a non-pitting facial edema characterized our case 6. The perilabial region of the 72-year-old patient was swollen; the pale skin was tense and the dermis seemed to be compact (Fig. 154). The biopsy specimen was taken from a blister-free area of the edematous skin.

Within the homogeneous upper dermis there were fewer elastic fibers (Fig. 155). In the middle and deep dermis the collagen fibers were arranged in large bundles running parallel with the epidermal surface. The dermal appendages were diminished. The lymphatic "lakes" localized in the reticular dermis were bordered by a flat endothelium surrounded by a poorly developed elastic network (Fig. 155).

Under the electron microscope the fragmented elastic fibers were situated apart from the abluminal endothelial cell membrane of the lymphatic capillaries. The collagen fibers varied between 20 and 80 nm in diameter and were embedded in an increased amount of granulofilamentous ground substance (Fig. 156). The lipid droplets discovered in the perivascular macrophages and in the endothelial cells are specific for chronic lymphedema (Fig. 157). Budding endothelial cells or valvular structures have rarely been seen in the lymphatic capillaries (Fig. 158).

19.2 Hyalinosis Cutis et Mucosae

This rare disorder is characterized by hyalin deposition involving the skin and the mucous membranes. Our 20-year-old female patient (case 7) had hoarseness due to infiltration of the vocal cord by hyalin and she complained about the vulnerability of her skin and superficial ulcers healing with scars. In addition chronic edema had developed on her face and neck (Fig. 159).

Histologically, the skin vessels and appendages were embedded in a massive coat of amorphous metachromatic material (Fig. 160). Seen under the electron microscope, the dermal vessels were wrapped in granulofilamentous material. The hyalin substance, consisting of basal lamina remnants, granular ground substance and collagen fragments, was arranged in concentric rings around the dermal vessels (Figs. 161 and 162). The basic morphological features of the lymphatic capillaries were not detectable (DARÓCZY and RÀCZ 1987).

19.3 Lichen Amyloidosus

Lichen amyloidosus belongs to the primary localized amyloidoses characterized by deposition of non-branching filaments measuring 10–15 nm in diameter in the subepidermal connective tissue. The usual form of the disease, as seen in our case 8, is localized on the stretching surface of the lower extremities and accompanied by a mild edema (Fig. 163).

Histologically, accumulation of the dye Congo red in the deposited amyloid substance and positive birefringence under the polarization microscope are diagnostic (Figs. 164 and 165). Under the electron microscope filamentous amyloid material can be seen to envelop both the blood and the lymphatic dermal capillaries. The elastic and collagen fibers were parted from the lymphatic endothelium by bundles of filaments measuring 10–12 nm in diameter and connected directly with the abluminal surface of the lymphatic endothelial cells (Figs. 166 and 167).

Porphyria cutanea tarda (case 6), hyalinosis cutis et mucosae (case 7), and lichen amyloidosus (case 8) are characterized by disturbances and remodeling of the dermal connective tissue through the deposit of substances of different origins. These cases call attention to the fact that the deposited substances occupy both the perivascular and perilymphatic spaces. Therefore, all clinical cases associated with lymphedema should be examined for an underlying lymphatic disturbance. Symptomatic treatment of the lymphedema may have a beneficial influence on the basic disorders.

Fig. 154. Porphyria cutanea tarda in a 72-year-old female patient, case 6. The facial edema that hinders the patient in closing her mouth is non-pitting

Fig. 155. Case 6: In the subepidermal homogeneous connective tissue the number of elastic fibers is decreased. The lymphatic capillary *(L)* is dilated. Orcein, × 150

Fig. 156. Case 6: The lymphatic endothelial cytoplasm, containing numerous vesicles along both the luminal and abluminal membranes, is rich in microfilaments *(mf)*. The basal lamina *(Bl)* is discontinuous. Collagen fibers *(Co)* of varying diameter are embedded in an increased amount of granulofilamentous ground substance. *Lu,* Lymphatic lumen; × 7200

Fig. 157. Case 6: The lymphatic lumen *(star)* is very narrow. The endothelial cell contains lipid droplets *(Li)*. The perivascular space is characterized by bundles of thin collagen *(Co)* measuring 20–30 nm in diameter, and by collagen fibers running randomly through the granulofilamentous ground substance. The elastic fibers *(E)* are present at a large distance from the endothelium. × 2500

Fig. 158. Case 6: In some places the perilymphatic basal lamina *(Bl)* is prominent or a thick basal lamina-like material is present. The endothelial cell, budding into the lumen, contains bundles of microfilaments *(mf)*, dense granules *(g)*, and polyribosomes. Lu_{1-2}, Lymphatic lumina; × 2500

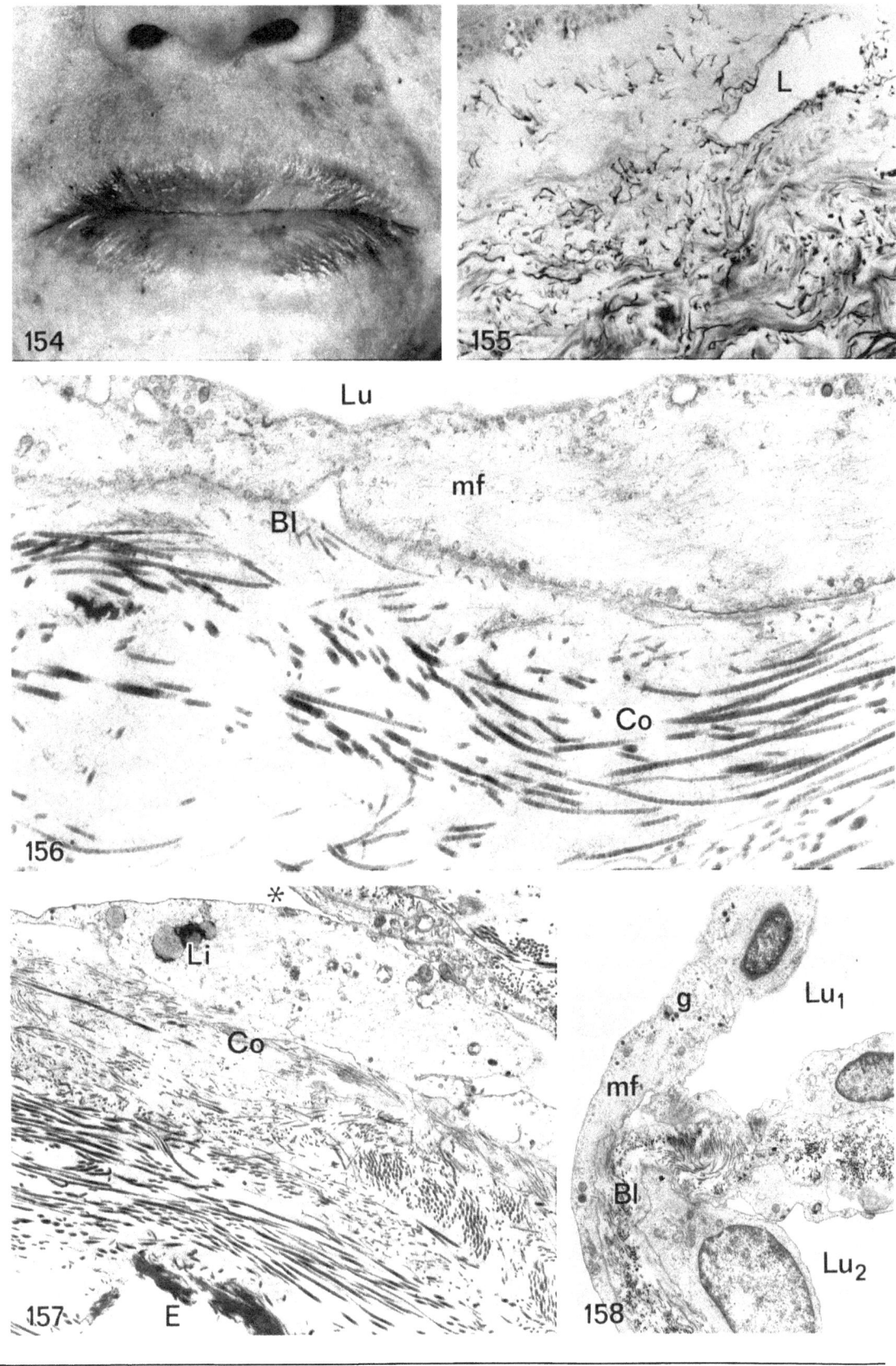

Fig. 159. Hyalinosis cutis et mucosae in a 20-year-old female patient, case 7. The lips, bordered by deep bleeding fissures and small waxy tumors along their inside margins, are swollen

Fig. 160. Case 7: The dermal vessels and appendages are surrounded by multiple concentric layers of homogeneous deposits in the connective tissue. Semithin section; toluidine blue, × 500

Fig. 161. The lumen *(Lu)* of the dermal vessel is lined by swollen endothelial cells containing dense mitochondria *(Mi)*. The pericytic layer is missing; the multiply folded basal lamina *(Bl)* material is intermingled with the granular ground substance. Some collagen fibers *(Co)* are embedded in the concentric shells of the connective tissue deposit. × 3500

Fig. 162. Elongated pseudopodia *(p)* of connective tissue cells and randomly arranged collagen fibers *(Co)* are embedded in the granulofilamentous substance of the connective tissue. The elastic fibers are diminished in number. × 5500

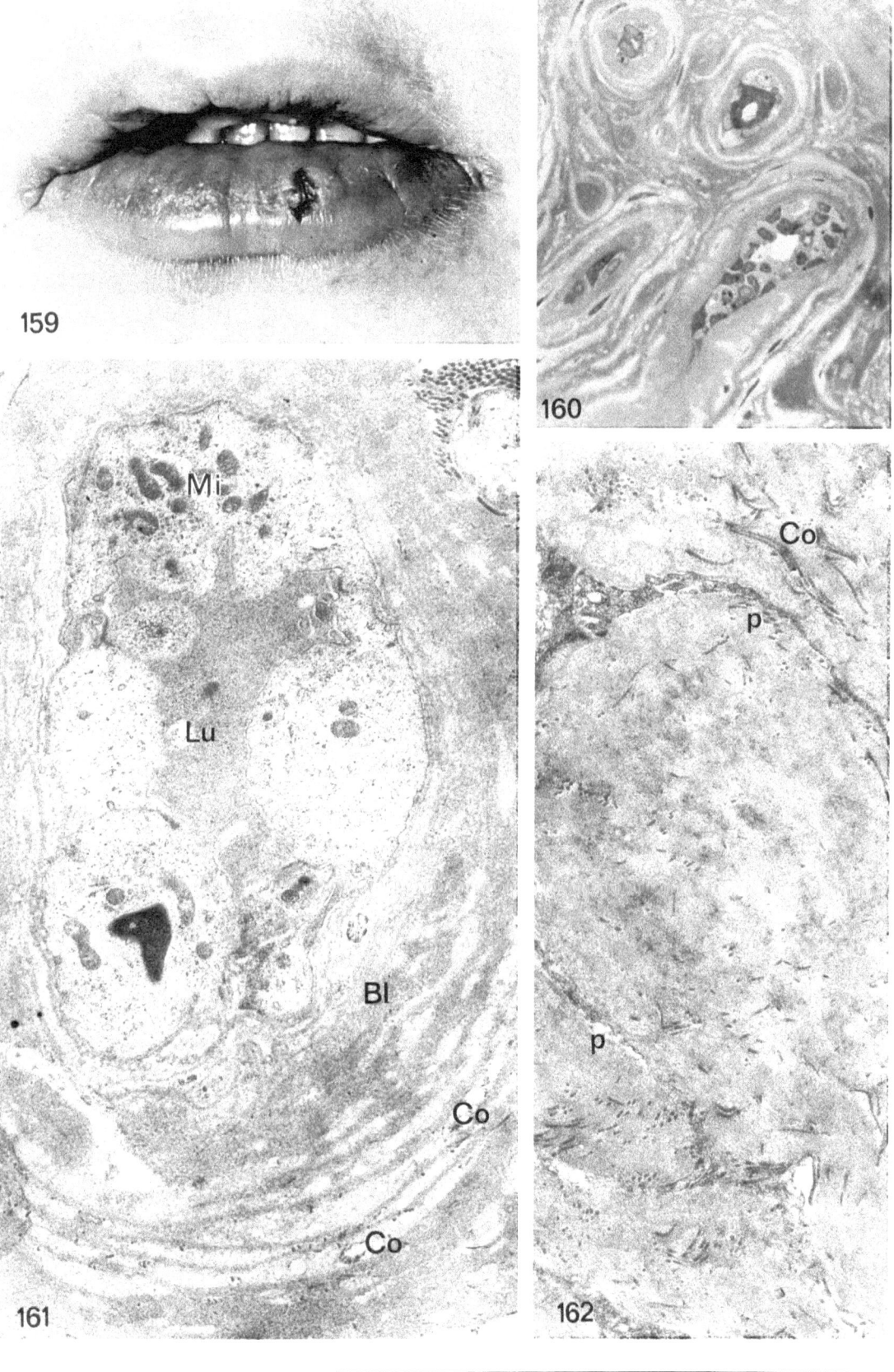

159

160

Mi

Lu

Bl

Co

Co

161

Co

p

p

162

Fig. 163. Lichen amyloidosus in a 42-year-old male patient, case 8. Shiny, waxy papules are seen over the left shin

Fig. 164. Case 8: The thick wall of a dilated dermal lymph vessel stained orange-red with Congo red. × 500

Fig. 165. Case 8: The same vessel as in Fig. 164 displays birefringence under polarized light. × 500

Fig. 166. Case 8: In the perivascular space of the lymphatic capillary the collagen fibers are intermingled with microfilaments *(f)* in increased numbers. The endothelial cell *(End)* surrounded by basal lamina-like material contains dense granules *(g)* and numerous microfilaments. The perivascular macrophage is loaded with lipid droplets *(Li)* and dense lysosomes. *Lu*, Lymphatic lumen; × 7200

Fig. 167. Case 8: The non-branching bundles of microfilaments *(f)*, 10–12 nm in diameter, running parallel with the long axis of the lymphatic capillary *(L)*, are accompanied by collagen *(Co)* and elastic *(E)* fibers. × 4000

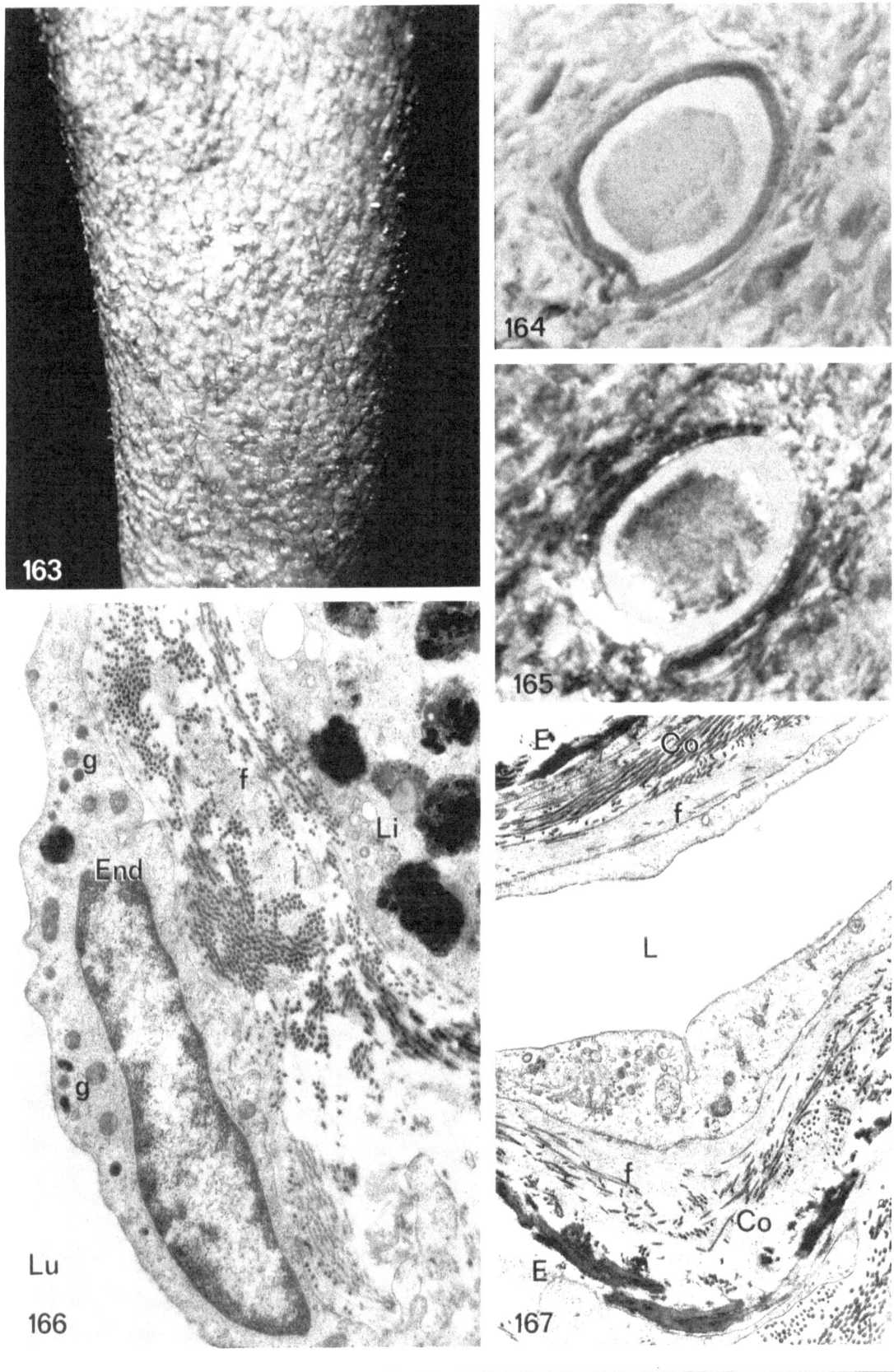

20 Lymphangitis

There is a high incidence of lymphangitis of the skin. The lymphatic vessels can reveal intact wall structures and are able to transport inflammatory cells from the infected dermal connective tissue without being affected themselves.

Lymphangitis can develop as a complication secondary to an inflammatory process. The infiltration involves the wall structures of the lymphatic vessel. Recurrent lymphangitis of the limbs following cutaneous microbial infections and recurrent episodes of erysipelas induce an obliterative lymphangitis, which can lead to fibrotic, irreversible lymphedema and to elephantiasis (BURKE and LEAK 1965; HUTH 1983).

Secondary lymphangitis has been found in connection with thrombophlebitis and thrombosis of the limbs. Fibrin thrombi have been documented in the lymphatics during experimental inflammation.

20.1 Lymphostatic Lymphangitis and Edema

In cutaneous and subcutaneous lymphangitis caused by recurrent infections the lymphatic capillaries are dilated. Granulocytic and plasmacellular infiltrates are detected in the lymphatic vessel walls and in the surrounding connective tissue. The endothelial cells are swollen. The congestion of the vessels and the inflammation can lead to an obliteration of the lymphatic lumina due to lymph thrombi.

20.2 Sclerosing Non-venereal Lymphangitis of the Penis

Non-venereal sclerosing lymphangitis of the penis manifests as a painless wormlike tender cord in the coronary sulcus which affects the dermal collecting lymphatic vessels. The lumen is occupied by fibrin thrombi which can be recanalized. The lumen is narrow, the vessel wall is fibrotic, and the fibroblasts are hypertrophic (KANDIL and AL-KASHLAN 1970; MARSCH and STÜTTGEN 1981).

20.3 Syphilis

Regional lymphadenitis connected with primary syphilitic infection is related to regional lymphangitis.

20.4 Parasitic Lymphangitis

HUTH (1983) distinguished lymphangitis following bacterial, viral, or parasitic infections from lymphangiosis characterized by the symptomatology of early reflux of lymph and the development of clincially perceptible lymphovascular funiculi.

Parasitic lymphangitis can occur in connection with schistosomiasis, ascariasis, echinococcosis, or trichinosis. Among the protozoal infections, leishmaniasis and trypanosomiasis have been reported with lymphovascular spreading of the parasites and pathological changes of the lymph vessel wall.

It is now clear that nematodes may propagate lymphovascularly. Histologically, lymphangiectasis, thromboangitis, chrombolymph-angitis, granulomatous proliferation, and fibrosis have been found. The pathogenesis of fibrotic edema is not quite understood. During filarial infestation with *Wuchereria bancrofti* the development of elephantoid edema of the limbs is relatively rare. In cases of filarial infestation by *Brugia malayi* there is a high incidence of elephantiasis of the lower limbs (DENHAM and McGREEVY 1977; TURNER 1959). Hypersensitivity to the infective agents and humoral and cellular immunolgical reactions play important roles in the pathogenesis of filarial lymphedema.

20.5 Lymphangitis in Mucormycosis

In subcutaneous mucormycosis, lymphovascular thrombi can serve as a medium for the growth of hyphae, causing destructive lymphangitis (HUTH 1983).

20.6 Lymphangitis due to Irritants

A form of lymphostatic elephantiasis without filariasis exists in Ethiopia. This form occurs after a transcutaneous absorption of aluminum silicate by the skin of the feet and after lymphovascular transport of the inorganic particles (HEATHER and PRICE 1972). Obliteration of the lymphatic vessels and lymph nodes is followed by lymphostatic edema.

The presence of silica and aluminum in the filtrating lymph node of the affected legs was evident by light- and electron-microscopical techniques and by emission spectroscopy (HUTH 1983). Aluminum silicate is an inhibitory factor in the connective tissue macrophages. This explains the development of lymphedema due to silica deposition in the dermal interstitium.

Another irritant is the contrast media used for radiological lymphangiography. These contrast materials can react with the endothelial cells of the perfused lymphatic vessels and the cells lining the lymphnode sinuses. The reaction around the drops of contrast medium can provoke a foreign-body granuloma with the formation of foam cells and multinucleated giant cells.

This reaction may lead to obliteration of the lymphatic lumen and sinuses; thus, latent lymphedema may become manifest after diagnostic lymphangiography.

20.7 Lymphangitis Carcinomatosa

Several studies have indicted the prognostic importance of peritumoral and blood vessel invasion. Standardized criteria for the recognition of abnormal vascularization are needed, as are pathologists who can identify these parameters. Such criteria have been developed for breast cancer, and an adverse prognostic significance of inflammatory peritumoral invasion of lymphatics was documented by NIME et al. (1977).

Increased and abnormal vascularization around skin tumors and melanomas have been detected, but a standardization of these probably prognostic signs is lacking.

In lymphangitis carcinomatosa tumor cells are detectable in the lymphatic lumen. These cancer cells continue to grow within the lumen in both directions. Dissemination of the cancer via the lymph vessels into the lymph nodes leads to the tumorous blockage of lymph node sinuses. Retrograde tumor extension can involve the lymphatic vessel wall, or the wall may be intact. The obstruction of the lymphatics and the blockage of the lymph nodes by the tumor cells cause a manifest peripheral edema.

Unilateral lymphedema was observed on the left lower limb of a patient suffering from lymphangitis carcinomatosa (case 9). On the left side of her lower abdominal wall and on her edematous left thigh solid funiculi and brownish papules were discovered 5 years after squamous cell carcinoma of the portio vaginalis uteri had been diagnosed (Figs. 168 and 169). The patient had refused any treatment.

The dermal lymphatics, accompanied by numerous monoculear inflammatory cells, contained large masses of tumor cells (Fig. 170).

Increased amounts of granulofilamentous ground substance and long-spacing collagen fibers were seen in the loose edematous environment of the dermal lymphatics (Fig. 171) under the electron microscope.

Fig. 168. Lymphangitis carcinomatosa in a 58-year-old female patient, case 9. The left lower limb is swollen due to secondary lymphedema. Skin papules are seen on the low abdominal wall and in the groin *(arrows)*

Fig. 169. Case 9: Close-up of the shiny brownish papules on the low abdominal wall

Fig. 170. Dilated dermal lymphatic capillary containing a mass of tumor cells is present in the vicinity of a dermal venule *(V)*. The edematous perivascular space is filled by mononuclear inflammatory cells. × 200

Fig. 171. Case 9: The perivascular space of the dermal vessels are characterized by a large amount of long-spacing collagen *(LSC)* and by increased granulofilamentous ground substance enveloping the collagen *(Co)* fibers. × 12000

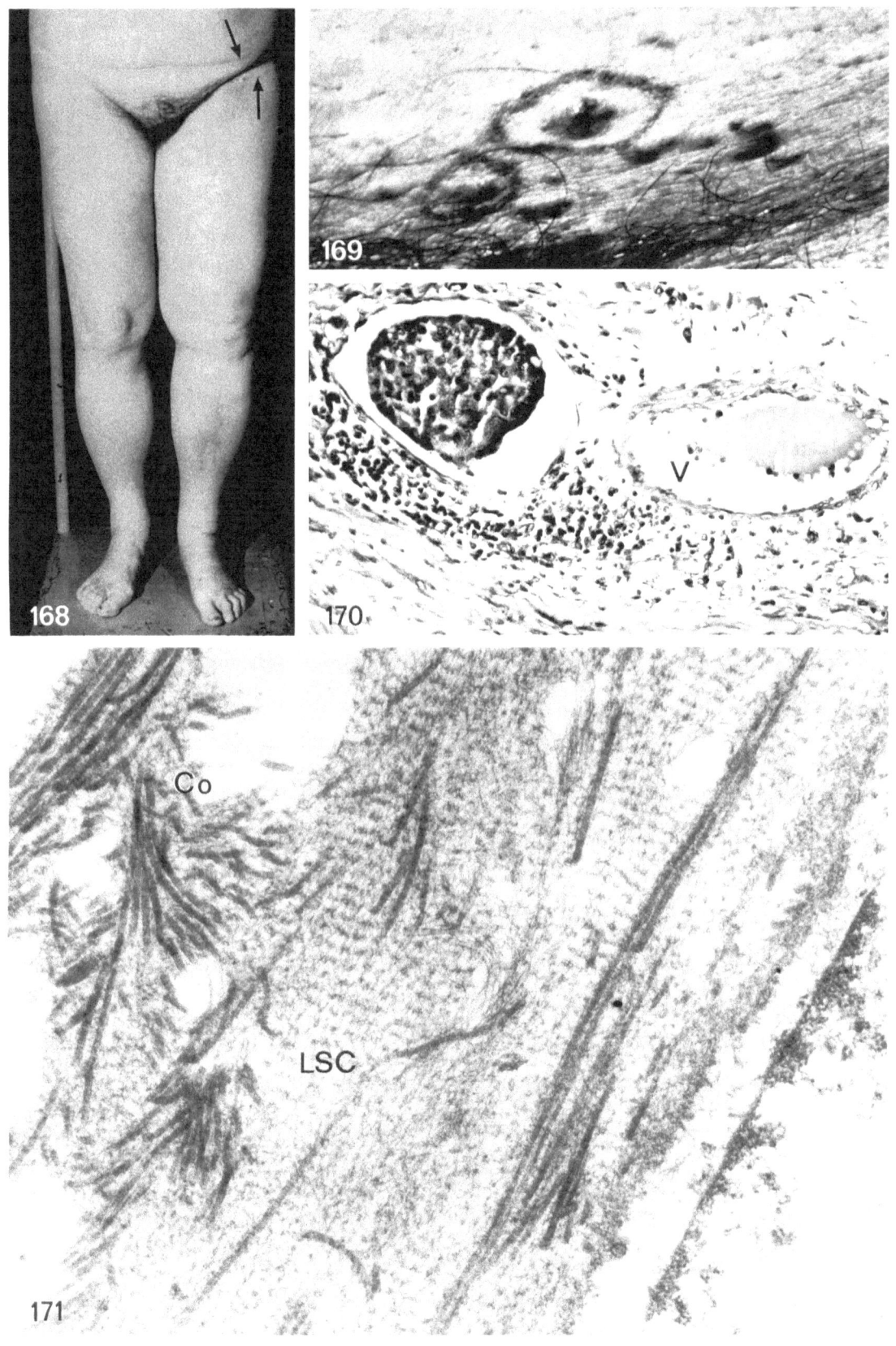

21 Treatment of Lymphostatic Edema

The three aims of treatment of lymphostatic edema are:

1. To remove the protein – to decrease protein content in the interstitium, to decrease osmotic pressure, and as a consequence to decrease the fluid volume (drug therapy)
2. To increase or maintain the lymphatic flow that removes large molecular substances (physical therapy)
3. To bypass the lymphatic block (surgery)

21.1 Drug Therapy

Macrophages digest protein and the protein fragments can pass into the blood vessels or venules via intercellular junctions and fenestrae. Benzopyrone (coumarin-5,6-benzo-alfa-pyron), pyridoxine, pantothenic acid, and complex vitamin-B components act by inducing incrased proteolysis of the extracellular proteins in the interstitium. Macrophages are believed to be the main cells affected by these drugs. The number of macrophages was increased in experimental animals treated with benzopyrone. The drug inhibits excess collagen formation (BOLTON and CASLEY-SMITH 1975).

Coumarin and benzopyrone proved to induce proteolysis and to increase the number of tranportable protein fragments in the connective tissue. These drugs have been shown to be very effective in reducing high-protein lymphedema (PILLER 1976a).

Benzopyrone administration has been observed to increase acid protease activities in the free edema fluid (PILLER 1976b). Electron-microscopical studies have shown that coumarin reduces protein concentration in both the lymphatics and the connective tissue (CASLEY-SMITH et al. 1973).

Coumarin does not increase the removal of non-metabolizable molecules (polyvinylpyrrolidine) and does not increase lymph flow.

Silicates are known to be selectively toxic for macrophages. The administration of silica prevents coumarin-stimualted lysis of accumulated protein. Coumarin was ineffecitve in reducing edema when experimental animals were injected with silicates that inactivated the proteolytic activity of macrophages.

Unguentum lymphaticum is a cream containing components (for example *Colchicum autumnale*, podophyllin, *Digitalis purpurea*) which have been shown to be effective in high-protein lymphedema in rats, produced by dextran and by burns. It would be preferable to investigate each of the pure components of the cream. It is supposed that the cream may act to increase proteolysis by macrophage induction. The cream is an inexpensive therapy (CASLEY-SMITH 1983).

Drug therapy is effective in lymphostatic edema, but it takes months to years to produce a good result.

21.2 Physical Therapy

The main forms of physical therapy are squeezing and massage. Manual or mechanically forced squeezing of the soft tissue is done with the aim of pressing the edematous fluid passively in a proximal direction. The apparatus used for this purpose are expensive and are insufficient in numerous clinical forms of edema. Application of pressure up to 75 mmHg to "wring out" the edematous fluid may traumatize the lymphatics.

Manual massage is progressively applicable; the technique is adaptable to the various clinical conditions, but it requires a physical thera-pist and a long uninterrupted period of treat-ment (i.e., many months).

The program of therapy must be completed with isometric muscle exercises and application of bandages over the treated limbs (FÖLDI et al. 1985; STIJNS and LEDUC 1977). Complex physi-cal therapy is usually excellent but it is expen-sive, involving a trained masseur. In one case of postmastectomy lymphedema a satisfactory ef-fect of the regional sympathetic block was demonstrated (SWEDBORG et al. 1983).

21.3 Surgical Therapy

In selected cases a surgical ablative procedure can be effective. There are two main types of operations. The first is surgical procedures *to increase lymph drainage,* i.e., to create lymphati-covenous shunts. The new drainage pathways bypass the blocked area. The creation of direct lymphaticovenous anastomoses requires special microsurgical equipment (CLODINS 1977; DE-GANI 1978). The aim of the second type of op-eration is to remove as much of the swollen fi-brotic subcutaneous tissue as possible.

References

Aboul-Enein H, Eshmawy I, Arafa S, Abboud A (1984) The role of lymphaticovenous communication in the development of postmastectomy lymphedema. Surgery 95: 562–566

Albertine KH, Fox LM, O'Morchoe CC (1980) Lymphatic endothelial cell inclusion bodies. J Ultrastruct Res 73: 199–210

Allen EV (1934) Lymphedema of the extremities: classification, etiology and differential diagnosis; a study of three hundred cases. Arch Intern Med 54: 606–624

Altorfer J, Clodins L (1976) Chronic experimental lymphedema of the extremities pathological changes. Experientia 32: 823–825

Armenio S, Cetta F, Tanzini G, Guercia C (1981) Spontaneous contractility in the human lymph vessels. Lymphology 14: 173–178

Asano S, Endo H, Sagami S (1978) An ultrastructural study of localized lymphangioma circumscriptum. Arch Dermatol Res 262: 301–309

Azuma T, Ohhashi T, Roddie LC (1983) Bradykinin-induced contraction of bovine mesenteric lymphatics. J Physiol 342: 217–227

Azzali G (1982) The ultrastructural basis of lipid transport in the absorbing lymphatic vessel. J Submicrosc Cytol 14: 45–54

Barker CF, Billingham RE (1968) The role of afferent lymphatics in the rejection of skin homografts. J Exp Med 128: 197–221

Bean WB (1955) Dyschondroplasia and Hemangiomata (Mafucci's syndrome Arch intern Med 95: 767–778

Beckstead JH, Wood GS, Fletcher V (1985) Evidence for the origin of Kaposi's sarcoma from lymphatic endothelium. Am J Pathol 119: 294–300

Bollinger A, Jajer K, Spier F, Seglias J (1981) Fluorescence microlymphangiography. Circulation 64: 1193–1198

Bolton T, Casley-Smith JR (1975) An in vitro demonstration of proteolysis by macrophages and its increase with coumarin. Experientia 31: 271–272

Braverman IM (1983) The role of blood vessels and lymphatics in cutaneous inflammatory processes: an overview. Br J Dermatol 109: 89–98

Braverman IM, Yen A (1974) Microcirculation in psoriatic skin. J Invest Dermatol 62: 493–502

Brunner U (1972) Zur Frühdiagnose des primären Lymphoedems der Beine. Vasa 1: 293–302

Burke JF, Leak LV (1965) Ultrastructure of lymphatic capillaries during the inflammatory response. J Cell Biol 27: 129A–130A

Casley-Smith JR (1964a) An electron-microscopic study of injured and abnormally permeable lymphatics. Ann NY Acad Sci 116: 803–830

Casley-Smith JR (1964b) Endothelial permeability – the passage of particles into and out of diaphragmatic lymphatics. Q J Exp Physiol 49: 365–383

Casley-Smith JR (1965) Endothelial permeability. II. The passage of particles through the lymphatic endothelium of normal and injured ears. Br J Exp Pathol 46: 34–49

Casley-Smith JR (1967) Electron-microscopical observations on the dilated lymphatics in edematous regions and their collapse following hyaluronidase administration. Br J Exp Pathol 48: 680–689

Casley-Smith JR (1979) A fine-structural study of variations in protein concentration in lacteals during compression and relaxation. Lymphology 12: 59–65

Casley-Smith JR (1983) The effect of "unguentum lymphaticum" on acute experimental lymphedema and other high-protein edemas. Lymphology 16: 150–156

Casley-Smith JR, Florey HW (1961) The structure of normal small lymphatics. Q J Exp Physiol 46: 101–107

Casley-Smith JR, Sims MA (1976) Protein concentrations in regions with fenestrated and continuous blood capillaries and in initial and collecting lymphatics. Microvasc Res 12: 245–257

Casley-Smith JR, Földi M, Zoltán ÖT (1969) The treatment of acute lymphedema with pantothenic acid and pyridoxine: an electron-microscopical investigation. Lymphology 2: 63–71

Casley-Smith JR, Földi-Börcsök, Földi M (1973a) The electron microscopy of the effects of treatment with coumarin (Venolot) and by thoracic duct cannulation of thermal injuries. Br J Exp Pathol 54: 1–5

Casley-Smith JR, Bolto T (1973b) Electron microscopy of the effects of histamine and thermal injury on the blood and lymphatic endothelium, and the mesothelium of the mouse diaphragm, together with the influence of coumarin and rutin. Experientia 29: 1386–1388

Castenholz A (1986) Die Lymphbahn im rasterelektromikroskopischen Bild. Ödem 1: 32–38

Clodius L (1977) Secondary arm lymphedema. In: Clodius L (ed) Lymphedema. Thieme, Stuttgart, pp 147–174

Collan Y, Kalima TV (1974) Topographical relations of lymphatic endothelial cells in the initial lymphatics of the intestine. Lymphology 7: 175–184

Colver GB, Ryan TJ (1983) Metachromatic cells in filarial lymphedema. Lancet II: 1248

Cornillie FJ, Lauweryns JM (1984) Fluid and protein clearance in the rat endometrium. II. Ultrastructural evidence for the presence of alternative, non-lymphatic clearance mechanism in the rat endometrium. Experientia 40: 1264–1266

Daróczy J (1982) Ultrastructure of dermal lymph capillaries in relation to their function. Verh Anat Ges 76: 347–348

Daróczy J (1983a) Die Struktur und Funktion der Klappen der dermalen Lymphkapillaren. Hautarzt 33: 136–138

Daróczy J (1983 b) Valve-mechanism and lock-gate chamber function of the dermal lymph vessels. J Cutan Pathol 10: 286

Daróczy J (1983 c) The structure and dynamic function of the dermal lymphatic capillaries. Br J Dermatol 109: 99–102

Daróczy J (1984 a) Die Struktur der dermalen Lymphkapillaren und ihre funktionelle Interpretation. Hautarzt 35: 630–639

Daróczy J (1984 b) New structural details of dermal lymphatic valves and their functional interpretation. Lymphology 17: 54–60

Daróczy J (1984 c) Functional interpretation of the structural characteristics of the dermal lymphatics. Int J Microcirc 3: 369

Daróczy J (1986) Pathologische Veränderungen der Lymphkapillarwand in Ödem. Ödem 1: 133–136

Daróczy J (1987) and Ràcz I. (1987) Diagnostic electron microscopy in practical dermatology. Akadémiai Kiadó, Budapest

Daróczy J, Hüttner I (1978) Fenestrated capillaries in the rat paw dermis adjacent to epidermis and skin appendages. Z Mikrosk Anat Forsch 92: 598–606

Degani U (1978) New technique of lymphaticovenous anastomosis for the treatment of lymphedema. J Cardiovasc Surg (Torino) 19: 577

Denham DA, McGreevy PA (1977) Brugian filariasis: epidemiological and experimental studies. Adv Parasitol 15: 244–309

DiLeonardo M, Jacoby RA (1986) Acquired cutaneous lymphangiectasias secondary to scarring from scrofuloderma. J Am Acad Dermatol 14: 688–690

Dobbins WO, Rollins EL (1970) Intestinal mucosal lymphatic permeability: an electron-microscopic study of endothelial vesicles and cell junctions. J Ultrastruct Res 33: 29–59

Dorman RF (1984) The histogenesis of Kaposi's sarcoma. Lymphology 17: 76–77

Dumont AE, Fazzini E, Jamal S (1983) Metachromatic cells in filarial lymphedema. Lancet II/II: 1021

Earhart RN, Aeling JA, Nuss DD, Mellette RJ (1974) Pseudo-Kaposi's sarcoma. Arch Dermatol 110: 907–910

Elfvin LG (1965) The ultrastructure of the capillary fenestrae in the adrenal medulla of the rat. J Ultrastruct Res 12: 687–704

Ellis JP, Marks R, Perry J (1970) Lymphatic function: the disappearance rate of [131]-I. Albumin from the dermis. Br J Dermatol 82: 593–599

Fischer I, Orkin M (1970) Acquired lymphangioma (lymphangiectasia). Arch Dermatol 101: 230–234

Flanagan BP, Helwig EB (1977) Cutaneous lymphangioma. Arch Dermaol 113: 24–30

Földi M (1969) Diseases of lymphatics and lymph circulation. Akadémiai Kiadó, Budapest

Földi M (1983) Lymphedema. In: Földi M, Casley-Smith JR (eds) Lymphangiology. Schattauer, Stuttgart, p 667

Földi E, Földi M, Weissleder H (1985) Conservative treatment of lymphedema of the limbs. Angiology 36: 171–180

Gange RW, Wilson-Jones E (1979) Lymphangioma-like Kaposi's sarcoma. Br J Dermatol 100: 327–334

Girard C, Johnson WC, Graham JM (1970) Cutaneous lymphangiosarcoma. Cancer 26: 868–883

Gnepp DR (1976) The bicuspid nature of the valves of the peripheral collecting lymphatic vessels of the dog. Lymphology 9: 75–77

Grimley PM, Schaff Z (1976) Significance of tubuloreticular inclusions in the pathobiology of human diseases. Pathobiol Ann 6: 221–257

Guyton AC (1963) A concept of negative interstitial pressure based on pressures in implanted perforated capsules. Circ Res 12: 399–414

Guyton AC, Coleman TG (1968) Regulation of interstitial fluid volume and pressure. Ann NY Acad Sci 150: 537–547

Heather CJ, Price EW (1972) Non-filarial elephantiasis in Ethiopia. Analytical study of inorganic material in lymph nodes. Trans R Soc Trop Med Hyg 66: 450–458

Heuvel NV, Stolz E, Notowicz A (1979) Lymphangiectasis of the vulva in patient with lymph node tuberculosis. Int J Dermatol 18: 65–66

Hiller E, Rosenow EC, Elsen AM (1972) Pulmonary manifestations of the yellow nail syndrome. Chest 61: 652–658

Hogan RED, Nicoll PA (1979) Quantitation of convective forces active in lymph formation. Microvasc Res 17: 145

Holbrook KA, Byers PH (1982) Structural abnormalities in the dermal collagen and elastic matrix from the skin of patients with inherited connective tissue disorders. J Invest Dermatol 79 [Suppl 1]: 7–16

Holden AC, Spaull J, Williams R, Spry CJ, Russel-Jones R, Wilson-Jones F (1986) The detection of endothelial cell antigens in cutaneous tissue using methacarn and periodate lysine paraformaldehyde fixation. J Immunol Methods 91: 45–52

Huth F (1983) General pathology of the lymphovascular system. In: Földi M, Casley-Smith JR (eds) Lymphangiology. Casley-Smith Schattauer, Stuttgart, pp 215–334

Johnston MG, Gordon JL (1981) Regulation of lymphatic contractility by arachidonate metabolites. Nature 293: 294–297

Johnston MG, Kanalec A, Gordon JL (1983) Effects of arachidonic acid and its cyclo-oxygenase and lipoxygenase products on lymphatic vessel contractility in vitro. Prostaglandins 25: 85–98

Jones WR, O'Morchoe PJ, O'Morchoe CCC (1983) The organization of endocytotic vesicles in lymphatic endothelium. Microvasc Res 25: 286–299

Jones RR, Spaull J, Spry SJ, Wilson Jones E (1986) The histogenesis of Kaposi's sarcoma in patients with and without AIDS. J Clin Pathol 39: 742–749

Kandil E, Al-Kashlan IM (1970) Non-veneral sclerosing lymphangitis of the penis. Acta Derm Venereol (Stockh) 50, 309–312

Karnovsky MJ (1965) A formaldehyde-glutaraldehyde fixative of high osmolality for use in electron microscopy. J Cell Biol 27: 137 a

King DT, Duffy DM, Hirose FM, Gurevitch AW (1979) Lymphangiosarcoma arising from lymphangioma circumscriptum. Arch Dermatol 115: 969–972

Kinmonth JB (1952) Lymphangiography in man. A method of outlining lymphatic trunks at operation. Clin Sci 11: 13–20

Kinmonth JB, Taylor GW (1956) Spontaneous rhythmic contractility in human lymphatics. J Physiol 133: 3

Kubik I, Szabó J (1955) Die Innervation der Lymphgefäße im Mesenterium. Acta Morphol Acad Sci Hung 6: 25–32

Kuo T, Gomez LG (1979) Papillary endothelial proliferation in cystic lymphangiomas. Arch Pathol Lab Med 103: 306–308

Lambert PB, Frank HA, Bellman S, Farnsworth D (1965) The role of the lymph trunks in the response to allogenic skin transplants. Transplantation 3: 62–73

Larsson E, Westermark P (1978) Chronic hypertrophic vulvitis – a condition wiht similarities to cheilitis granulomatosa (Melkersson-Rosenthal syndrome). Acta Derm Venereol (Stockh) 58: 92–93

Laskas JJ, Shelley WB, Wood MG (1975) Lymphangiosarcoma arising in congenital lymphedema. Arch Dermatol 111: 86–89

Lauweryns JJ (1971) Stereomicroscopic funnel-like architecture of pulmonary lymphatic valves. Lympholgoy 4: 125

Lauweryns JM, Cornillie FJ (1984) Fluid and protein clearance in the rat endometrium. I. Ultrastructural proof of the absence of an intrinsic lymphatic system from the rat endometrium. Experientia 40: 1262–1264

Leak LV (1971) Studies on the permeability of lymphatic capillaries. J Cell Biol 50: 300–323

Leak LV (1972a) The transport of exogenous peroxidase across the blood-tissue-lymph interface. J Ultrastruct Res 39: 24–42

Leak LV (1972b) The fine structure and function of the lymphatic vascular system. In: Meessen H (ed) Lymphgefäß-System, Handbuch der allgeimen Pathologie. Springer, Berlin Heidelberg New York, pp 149–196

Leak LV (1976) The structure of lymphatic capillaries in lymph formation. Fed Proc 35: 1863–1871

Leak LV, Burke JF (1968) Ultrastructural studies on the lymphatic anchoring filaments. J Cell Biol 36: 129–149

Leak LV, Kato F (1972c) Electron-microscopic studies of lymphatic capillaries during early inflammation. Lab Invest 26: 572–588

Lehmann HD (1983) Pharmacology of the lymphatics. In: Földi M, Casley-Smith JR (eds) Lymphangiology. Schattauer, Stuttgart, pp 707–721

Lindemayr W, Lofferer O, Mostbeck A, Partsch H (1984) Neue Aspekte in der Diagnostik venöser und lymphathischer Erkrankungen der Beine. Z Hautkr 59: 1013–1023

Lynde CW, Mitchell JC (1982) Unusual complication of allergic contact dermatitis of the hands – recurrent lymphangitis and persistent lymphedema. Contact Dermatitis 8: 279–280

Mahzoon S, Azadeh B (1983) Elephantiasis of external ears: a rare manifestation of pediculosis capitis. Acta Derm Venereol (Stockh) 63: 363–365

Malek P (1972) Lymphaticovenous anastomoses. In: H. Meessen (ed) Lymphgefäß-System, Handbuch der allgemeinen Pathologie, vol. 3. Springer, Berlin Heidelberg New York, pp 197–218

Mali JWH, Kuiper JP, Hamers AA (1965) Acroangiodermatitis of the foot. Arch Dermatol 92: 515–518

Mannheimer E, Sinzinger H, Oppolzer R, Silberbauer K (1980) Prostacyclin synthesis in human lymphatics. Lymphology 13: 44–46

Marsch WC, Stüttgen G (1981) Sclerosing lymphangitis of the penis: a lymphangiofibrosis thrombotica occlusiva. Br J Dermatol 104: 687–695

May R, Nissl R (1970) Beitrag zur Klassifizierung der "gemischten kongenitalen Angiodysplasien". Fortschr Roentgenstr 113: 170–175

McHale NG, Allen JM (1983) The effect of external Ca^{2+} concentration on the contractility of bovine mesenteric lymphatics. Microvasc Res 26: 182–192

McHale NG, Roddie IC (1976) The effect of transmural pressure on pumping activity in isolated bovine lymphatic vessels. J Physiol 261: 255–269

McHale NG, Roddie IC, Thornbury KD (1980) Nervous modulation of spontaneous contractions in bovine mesenteric lymphatics. J Physiol 309: 461–472

McMaster PD (1946) The pressure and interstitial resistance prevailing in the normal and edematous skin of animals and man. J Exp Med 84: 473

McNutt NS, Fletcher V, Conant MA (1983) Early lesions of Kaposi's sarcoma in homosexual men. Am J Pathol 111: 62–77

Melkersson E (1928) Ett fall av recidiverande fasialisparese i samband med angioneurotiskt ödem. Hygiea (Stockholm) 90: 737–741

Mischer G (1945) Über essentielle granulomatöse Makrocheilie (Cheilitis granulomatosa). Dermatologica 91: 57–85

Mislin H (1961) Experimenteller Nachweis der autochthonen Automatie der Lymphgefäße. Experientia 17: 29–30

Mislin H (1976) Active contractility of the lymphangion and coordination of lymphangion chains. Experientia 32: 820–822

Mortimer PS, Ryan TJ (1986) Lymphoedema. Lancet I: 688–689

Mortimer PS, Cherry GW, Jones RL, Barnhill RL, Ryan TJ (1983) The importance of elastic fibers in skin lymphatics. Br J Dermatol 108: 561–566

Mukai K, Rosai J, Burgdork WHC (1980) Localization of factor VIII-related antigen in vascular endothelial cells using an immunoperoxidase method. Am J Surg Pathol 4: 273

Nicoll PA, Taylor AE (1977) Taylor Lymph formation and flow. Ann Rev Physiol 39: 73–95

Nime FA, Rosen PP, Thaler HT (1977) Prognostic significance of tumor emboli in intramammary lymphatics in patients. Am J Surg Pathol 1: 25–29

Nishida S, Ohkuma M (1983) Enzyme-histochemical differentiation of the human cutaneous lymphatic from the blood capillary. Immunol Hematol Res 2: 108–113

Oehmke HJ (1968) Periphäre Lymphgefäße des Menschen und ihre funktionelle Struktur. Z Zellforsch 90: 320–332

Ohhashi T, Azuma T (1984) Variegated effects of prostaglandins on spontaneous activity in bovine mesenteric lymphatics. Microvasc Res 27: 71–80

Ohhashi T, Azuma T, Sakaguchi M (1980) Active and passive mechanical characteristics of bovine mesenteric lymphatics. Am J Physiol 239: H88–95

Ohkuma M (1979) Histochemical change of the endothelial basal lamina of the diabetic lymphatic vessel. Lymphology 12: 37–39

Ohkuma M (1982) Lymphatics of the skin. Proc 8th Int. Congress of Lymphology, Montreal, 1981. Avicenum, Czechoslowak Medical press, Prague, pp 84–92

Olszewski W (1977) Pathophysiological and clinical observations of obstructive lymphedema of the limbs. In: Clodins L (ed) Lymphedema. Thieme, Suttgart, pp 79–102

O'Morchoe PJ, Yang VV, O'Morchoe CCC (1980) Lymphatic transport. Pathways during volume expansion. Microvasc Res 20: 275–294

Ottesen EA, Neva FA, Paranjape RS, Tripathy SP, Thiruvengadam KV, Beavan MA (1979) Specific allergic sensitisation to filarial antigens in tropical eosinophilia syndrome. Lancet 1 (8118): 1158–1161

Palade GE, Bruns RR (1968) Structural modulations of plasmalemmal vesicles. J Cell Biol 37: 633–649

Palmer LC, Strauch WG, Welton WA (1978) Lymphangioma circumscriptum. Arch Dermatol 114: 384–396

Papp M, Röhlich P, Rusznyák I, Törő I (1962) An electron-microscopic study of the central lacteal n the intestinal villus of the cat. Z Zellforsch Mikr Anat 57: 475–486

Partsch H, Wenzel-Hora BI, Urbanek A (1983) Differential diagnosis of lymphedema after indirect lymphangiography with iotasul. Lymphology 16: 12

Peachey RDG, Lim CC, Whimster IW (1970) Lymphangioma of skin. Br J Dermatol 83: 519–527

Pfleger L (1964 a) Histologie und Histopathologie kutaner Lymphgefäße der unteren Extremitäten. Arch Klin Exp Dermatol 221: 1–22

Pfleger L (1964 b) Histologie und Histopathologie kutaner Lymphgefäße der unteren Extremitäten. I. Morphologie der kutanen Lymphgefäße. Arch Klin Exp Deramtol 221: 23–58

Piller NB (1976 a) The ineffectiveness of coumarin treatment on thermal oedema of macrophage-free rats. Br J Exp Pathol 57: 170–178

Piller NB (1976 b) Drug-induced proteolysis: a correlation with oedema-reducing ability. Br J Exp Pathol 57: 266–273

Poggi P, Marchetti C, Calligaro A, Casasco A (1986) Cytoplasmic bodies in lymphatic endothelial cell. Lymphology 19: 125–129

Postacchini F, Sadun R (1976) Lymphangioma of the thigh following acute trauma. Clin Orthop Rel Res 121: 169–172

Pressman JJ, Dunn RF, Burtz M (1967) Lymph node ultrastructure related to direct lymphaticovenous communication. Surg Gynecol Obstet 124: 963–973

Pullinger BD, Florey HW (1935) Some observations on the structure and function of lymphatics: their behavior in local edema. Br J Exp Pathol 16: 49

Rajka Ö, Korossy S (1954) Neuroangiosis cruris haemosiderosa. The etiopathogenesis of "ulcus cruris" (in Hungarian). Orv Hetil 45: 57–63

Reed RJ, Palomeque FE, Hairston MA, Krementz ET (1966) Lymphangiosarcomas of the scalp. Arch Dermatol 94: 396–402

Roddie IC, Mawhinney HJ, McHale NG, Kirkpatrick CT, Thornbury K (1980) Lymphatic motility. Lymphology 13: 166–172

Rusznyák I, Földi M, Szabó G (1967) Lymphologie. Physiologie und Pathologie der Lymphgefäße und des Lymphkreislaufes. Fischer, Stuttgart

Rutgers JL, Wieczorek R, Bonetti, F et al. (1986) The expression of endothelial cell surface antigens by AIDS-associated Kaposi's sarcoma. Am J Pathol 122: 493–499

Ryan TJ, Mortimer PS, Jones RL (1986) Lymphatics of the skin. Int J Dermatol 25: 411–419

Samman PD, White WF (1964) The yellow nail syndrome. Br J Dermatol 76: 153–154

Schipp R (1968) Feinbau filamentärer Strukturen im Endothel peripherer Lymphgefäße. Acta Anat (Basel) 71: 341–351

Schlingemann RO, Dingjon GM, Emeis JJ, Blok J, Warnaar SO, Ruiter DJ (1985) Monoclonal antibody PAL-E specific for endothelium. Lab Invest 52: 71–76

Schmitz-Rixen T, Horsch S, Arnold G, Peters PE (1984) Angiosarkom beim primären Lymphödem der unteren Extremität – Stewart-Treves-Syndrom. Vasa 13: 262–266

Schneider I, Simon N, Zoltan ÖT, Földi M (1968) Veränderungen in der Haut des Halses beim Hunde nach Unterbindung der Lymphbahnen. Arch Klin Exp Dermatol 232: 367–372

Shea SM (1971) Lanthanum staining of the surface coat of cells. Its enhancement by the use of fixatives containing alcian blue or cetylpyridinium chloride. J Cell Biol 51: 611–620

Silverberg SG, Kay S, Koss LG (1971) Postmastectomy lymphangiosarcoma: ultrastructural observations. Cancer 27: 100–108

Simionescu N, Simionescu M, Palade GE (1975) Permeability of muscle capillaries to small hemipeptides. Evidence for the existence of patent transendothelial channels. J Cell Biol 64: 586–607

Sokolowski J, Jakobsen E, Johannessen JV (1978) Cells in peripheral leg lymph of normal men. Lymphology 11: 202–207

Solti F (1986) Personal discussion

Solti F, Ungváry G, Bálint A (1971) The regulation of the limb circulation in lymphoedema. Development of an arteriovenous shunt circulation in experimental lymphoedema. Angiologia 8: 117–124

Starling EH (1896) On the absorption of fluids from the connective tissue spaces. J Physiol (Lond) 19: 312–326

Stemmer R (1976) Ein klinisches Zeichen zur Früh- und Differentialdiagnose des Lymphödems. Vasa 5: 261–262

Stewart FW, Treves N (1948) Lymphangiosarcome in postmastectomy lymphedema. A report of six cases of elephantiasis chirurgica. Cancer 1: 64–81

Stijns HJ, Leduc A (1977) The contribution of physical therapy in the treatment of lymphedema. In: Clodins L (ed) Lymphedema. Thieme, Stuttgart, pp 27–32

Storrs TJ (1975) The Melkersson-Rosenthal syndrome. Br J Oral Surg 13: 160–165

Svanholm H, Nielsen K, Hange P (1984) Factor VIII-related antigen and lymphatic collecting vessels. Virchows Arch [A] 404: 223–228

Swedborg I, Arnér S, Meyerson BA (1983) New approaches to sympathetic blocks as treatment of postmastectomy lymphedema. Lymphology 16: 157–163

Szabó G, Magyar Z (1967) Pressure measurement in various parts of the lymphatic system. Acta Med Acad Sci Hung 23: 237–241

Szegvári M, Lakos A, Szontágh F, Földi M (1963) Spontaneous contractions of lymphatic vessels in man. Lancet I: 1329

Szegvári M, Lakos A, Szontágh F, Földi M (1964) The active function of the subcutaneous lymphatic vessels of the human lower extremity. Acta Med Acad Sci Hung 20: 209–213

Takada M (1971) The ultrastructure of lymphatic valves in rabbits and mice. Am J Anat 132: 207–218

Taylor AE, Gibson WH, Granger HS, Guyton AC (1973) The interaction between intracapillary and tissue forces in the overall regulation of interstitial fluid volume. Lymphology 6: 192–212

Threefoot SA, Kossover MF (1966) Lymphaticovenous communications in man. Arch Int Med 117: 213–223

Töndury G and Kubik St (1972) Zur Ontogenese des lymphatischen Systems. In: Handbuch der Allgmeinen Pathologie, Vol. III. Springer, Berlin, Heidelberg New York pp 1–38

Turner LH (1959) Studies on filariasis in Malaga. Trans R Soc Trop Med Hyg 53: 154–169

Vajda J (1966) Innervation of lymph vessels. Acta Morphol Acad Sci Hung 14: 197–208

Vajda J, Tomcsik M (1971) The structure of the valves of the lymphatic vessels. Acta Anat 78: 521–531

Virágh S, Papp M, Törő I, Rusznyák I (1966) Cutaneous lymphatic capillaries in dextran-induced oedema of the rat. Br J Exp Pathol 47: 563–567

Vogel A (1972) The pharmacology of the lymph and the lymphatic system. In: Meessen H (ed) Lymphgefäß-System. Handbuch der Allgemeinen Pathologie, vol 3. Springer, Berlin Heidelberg New York, pp 363–404

Weakley DR, Juhlin EA (1961) Lymphangiectases and lymphangiomata. Arch Dermatol 84: 574–578

Weibel EP, Palade GE (1964) New cytoplasmic components in arterial endothelia. J Cell Biol 23: 101

Whimster IW (1976) The pathology of lymphangioma circumscriptum. Br J Dermatol 94: 473–486

Worm AM, Staberg B, Thomsen K (1983) Persistent oedema in allergic contact dermatitis. Contact Dermatitis 9: 517–518

Yang VV, O'Morchoe PJ, O'Morchoe CCC (1981) Transport of protein across lymphatic endothelium in the rat kidney. Microvasc Res 21: 75–91

Yasuda A, Ohshima N (1984) In situ observations of spontaneous contractions of the peripheral lymphatic vessels in the rat mesentery. Effects of temperature. Experientia 40: 342–343

Zerbino DD (1960) Altersveränderungen der efferenten lymphatischen Gefäße. Arch Anat Cistol Embryol (Strasb) 39: 37–42

Zsdanov DA (1952) Allgemeine Anatomie und Physiologie des Lymphgefäßsystem. Medgis, Leningrad

Zweifach BW (1973) Microcirculation. Ann Rev Physiol 35: 117–150

Subject Index